T0314251

A Research Agenda for COVID-19 and Society

Elgar Research Agendas outline the future of research in a given area. Leading scholars are given the space to explore their subject in provocative ways, and map out the potential directions of travel. They are relevant but also visionary.

Forward looking and innovative, Elgar Research Agendas are an essential resource for PhD students, scholars and anybody who wants to be at the forefront of research.

Titles in the series include

A Research Agenda for Manufacturing Industries in the Global Economy
Edited by John R. Bryson, Chloe Billing, William Graves and Godfrey Yeung

A Research Agenda for Global Higher Education
Jeroen Huisman and Marijk van der Wende

A Research Agenda for Real Estate
Edited by Piyush Tiwari and Julie T. Miao

A Research Agenda for Political Marketing
Edited by Bruce I. Newman and Todd P. Newman

A Research Agenda for Public–Private Partnerships and the Governance of Infrastructure
Edited by Graeme A. Hodge and Carsten Greve

A Research Agenda for Governance
John Pierre, B. Guy Peters, Jacob Torfing and Eva Sørensen

A Research Agenda for Sport Management
Edited by David Shilbury

A Research Agenda for COVID-19 and Society
Edited by Steve Matthewman

A Research Agenda for COVID-19 and Society

Edited by

STEVE MATTHEWMAN

Professor in Sociology, the School of Social Sciences | Te Puna Mārama, University of Auckland | Waipapa Taumata Rau, Aotearoa New Zealand

Elgar Research Agendas

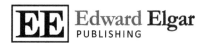

Edward Elgar
PUBLISHING

Cheltenham, UK • Northampton, MA, USA

Published by
Edward Elgar Publishing Limited
The Lypiatts
15 Lansdown Road
Cheltenham
Glos GL50 2JA
UK

Edward Elgar Publishing, Inc.
William Pratt House
9 Dewey Court
Northampton
Massachusetts 01060
USA

A catalogue record for this book
is available from the British Library

Library of Congress Control Number: 2022938796

This book is available electronically in the **Elgar**online
Sociology, Social Policy and Education subject collection
http://dx.doi.org/10.4337/9781800885141

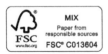

ISBN 978 1 80088 513 4 (cased)
ISBN 978 1 80088 514 1 (eBook)

Printed and bound by CPI Group (UK) Ltd, Croydon, CR0 4YY

Contents

Figures

Contributors

Marianne Clark is a postdoctoral fellow in the Vitalities Lab, Social Policy Research Centre and Centre for Social Research in Health, University of New South Wales, Sydney, Australia. Her work encompasses socio-cultural perspectives of the moving body and the role of digital technologies in shaping lived experiences and understandings of health.

Lyn Craig is professor and discipline chair of sociology, social policy and social theory, in the School of Social and Political Sciences, University of Melbourne, Australia. Her expertise includes the time impacts of children and care; intersections between the family and the economy; the gendered division of labour; and comparative family and social policy.

Tim Dare is professor of philosophy at the University of Auckland, Aotearoa, New Zealand. He worked briefly as a lawyer before doing his PhD in the philosophy of law and starting his academic career in the early 1990s. His publications include books and articles on the philosophy of law, legal ethics, immunisation programmes, parental rights and medical decisions, the proper allocation of the burden of proof and the use of predictive analytics in child protection. He provides research and operational ethics advice for several of New Zealand's government ministries and sits on a number of local and national research and clinical ethics committees.

Cordula Dittmer is a senior research assistant at the Disaster Research Unit (DRU), Freie University of Berlin, Germany; consultant at the Academy of Disaster Research (AKFS); and lecturer at the Berlin Fire and Rescue Academy. She holds a PhD in sociology with a focus on peace and conflict studies. She has conducted extensive field research on disasters in Uttarakhand, India, Northern Greece and Germany. Her publications and lectures explore, among other topics, theoretical and ethical aspects in social science disaster research, vulnerability and resilience and practices of dealing with disasters in disaster management organisations.

Luke Goode is associate professor and programme director for communication at the University of Auckland, Aotearoa New Zealand. His areas of research interest include: new and emerging communication technologies, communication and democracy and critical futures studies. His current obsession is the question of how we incorporate more constructive and hopeful modes of futures thinking into humanistic social science curricula and research agendas, without compromising on the vital work of critique and historicisation. He is one of the co-founding editors of the newly established *Journal of Social and Cultural Possibilities*.

Kate Huppatz is an associate professor of sociology, discipline lead and associate dean of research at the University of Western Sydney, Australia. She is interested in exploring the role of culture in the production and reproduction of inequalities and specialises in the study of gender, labour, education and households. Her forthcoming book is titled *Gender, Work and Social Theory* (Palgrave Macmillan).

Justine Kingsbury is a senior lecturer in philosophy and associate dean postgraduate of the Division of Arts, Law, Psychology and Social Sciences at the University of Waikato, Aotearoa New Zealand. Her areas of research include applied epistemology, philosophy of mind and aesthetics.

Simon Lambert is a Māori scholar who has worked in the Indigenous Disaster Risk Reduction (DRR) space since the 2011 earthquakes in Christchurch. His tribal affiliations are to Tūhoe and Ngāti Ruapani mai Waikaremoana. Since 2017 he has been based at the University of Saskatchewan, Canada, as an associate professor in Indigenous studies and is currently the executive director of the National Coordinating Centre of the Canadian federally funded Network Environments of Indigenous Health Research. He is also a member of the Pan-American Health Organization's Indigenous Knowledge and DRR Advisory Board.

Daniel F. Lorenz is a senior researcher at the Disaster Research Unit (DRU) at Freie Universität Berlin, Germany. Additionally, he coordinated projects for the Academy of the Disaster Research Unit (ADRU) and is lecturer of disaster research in a study program on emergency and crisis management. In 2017, he was a visiting researcher at the International Research Institute of Disaster Science (IRIDeS), Tohoku University, Sendai, Japan. He has conducted research in Germany, India, Japan, South Korea, Sierra Leone, Portugal and Greece, among other places. His research interests include various social science issues in the context of disasters and humanitarian emergencies such as social vulnerability and resilience.

Deborah Lupton is SHARP professor, member of the Centre for Social Research in Health and Social Policy Research Centre, leader of the Vitalities Lab and leader of the UNSW Node, leader of the Health Focus Area and co-leader of the People Program of the ARC Centre of Excellence for Automated Decision-Making and Society, all at the University of New South Wales, Sydney, Australia. An author/co-author of 18 books and editor–co-editor of a further nine volumes, her scholarship spans sociology, media studies and cultural studies.

Steve Matthewman is a professor in sociology at the University of Auckland, Aotearoa New Zealand. He is the immediate past president of the Sociological Association of Aotearoa New Zealand. Research interests include: communitas in disaster, the connections between resilience and vulnerability and the use of social capital to understand differential disaster outcomes. His current work focuses on the rebuilding of Christchurch following the 2010 and 2011 earthquakes. He is particularly interested in how a city gets put back together and what the barriers are to 'building back better'. His monograph *Disasters, Risks and Revelation: Making Sense of Our Times* was published in 2015. His latest edited collection is a book project on a decade of disasters in Canterbury, Aotearoa New Zealand, which will be published by Routledge.

Naoise McDonagh is a lecturer in the School of Economics and Public Policy at the University of Adelaide, Australia. He researches international political economy, institutional economics, and comparative capitalism, with specialisation in the macro evolution of economic systems. He has studied and worked in universities in Europe, New Zealand and Australia (current). Prior to entering academia, Naoise served two years in the Irish Defence Forces (2002–04) and worked in the private sector for five years (2004–09). He regularly publishes his research in internationally recognised journals, as well as leading policy forums such as the G20's annual Think 20 policy event. Research in progress analyses the political economy of WTO reform, the rise of geopolitical instability and its effect on trading relationships, the re-emergence of state-led capitalism and the growing role of state-owned enterprises in global trade.

Clare Southerton is a postdoctoral fellow in the Vitalities Lab, Social Policy Research Centre and Centre for Social Research in Health, University of New South Wales, Sydney, Australia. Her research explores the intersections between social media and digital technologies, and issues related to intimacy, sexuality, privacy and health.

Susanna Trnka is a professor of social anthropology at the University of Auckland. Her work focuses on citizen-state relations through the lenses of health and embodiment. She is the author of *Traversing: Embodied Lifeworlds in the Czech Republic* (Cornell University Press, 2020), *One Blue Child: Asthma, Responsibility and the Politics of Global Health* (Stanford University Press, 2017) and *State of Suffering: Political Violence and Community Survival* *in Fiji* (Cornell University Press, 2008). In addition to her work on COVID-19, she is currently running a multi-disciplinary research project examining digital technology use and youth mental health.

Deborah Wallace received her PhD in symbiosis ecology from Columbia University in 1971. In 1972, she became an environmental studies manager at Consolidated Edison Co. and participated in pioneering environmental impact assessment. She became a manager of biological and public health studies at NYS Power Authority in 1974 and remained there until early 1982. In 1980 she completed a mini residency in epidemiology at Mt. Sinai Medical Center. In the mid-1970s, she also founded Public Interest Scientific Consulting Service which produced impact assessments of massive cuts in fire service in New York City. She also probed the health threats that plastics in fires posed to firefighters and became an expert witness in litigation for plaintiffs in large fires fuelled by plastics. From 1985–1991, she worked for Barry Commoner at the Center for the Biology of Natural Systems at Queens College. During 1991–2010, she tested consumer products and services for their environmental and health impacts at Consumers Union. She retired in 2010 but continues data analysis, research and scientific publications. Her first paper was published in 1975, and her latest publication, a book on COVID-19 in New York, in 2020.

Rodrick Wallace is a research scientist in the Division of Epidemiology at the New York State Psychiatric Institute, affiliated with Columbia University's Department of Psychiatry, in the United States of America. He has an undergraduate degree in mathematics and a PhD in physics from Columbia, and completed postdoctoral training in the epidemiology of mental disorders at Rutgers. He worked as a public interest lobbyist, including two decades conducting empirical studies of fire service deployment, and subsequently received an Investigator Award in Health Policy Research from the Robert Wood Johnson Foundation. In addition to material on public health and public policy, he has published peer reviewed studies modelling evolutionary process and heterodox economics, as well as many quantitative analyses of institutional and machine cognition. He publishes in the military science literature, and in 2019 received one of the UK MoD RUSI Trench Gascoigne Essay Awards.

Ash Watson is a postdoctoral fellow with the ARC Centre of Excellence for Automated Decision-Making and Society, based at the University of New South Wales, Sydney, Australia. She is a sociologist of technology, fiction and DIY community practices.

L.L. Wynn is associate professor in the School of Social Sciences (discipline of anthropology) at Macquarie University in Sydney, Australia and president emerita of the Australian Anthropological Society. She is the author of two monographs, *Pyramids and Nightclubs* (University of Texas Press, 2007) and *Love, Sex, and Desire in Modern Egypt: Navigating the Margins of Respectability* (University of Texas Press, 2018). She has also co-edited three books, the most recent of which is *Sex in the Middle East and North Africa* (Vanderbilt University Press, in press for 2022). Her research on COVID-19 is supported by grants from the Social Science Research Council and the Australian Research Council.

Richey Wyver teaches sociology at the University of Auckland, Aotearoa New Zealand. His current research relates to questions of Swedish whiteness and perceptions of Swedishness, particularly in relation to international adoption. His doctoral thesis, *'More Beautiful than Something We Could Create Ourselves': Exploring Swedish International Adoption Desire* entailed a critical study of Sweden's role in the international adoption industry, and explored how transracial adoptees are used in constructing images of Swedish 'goodness', and in concealing the violence of Sweden's racist and colonial past and present. Richey lived in Sweden for several years, completing BA and MA degrees in international migration and ethnic relations at Malmo University.

Acknowledgements

The editor would like to thank Professor Ruth Fitzgerald, University of Otago, for permitting reproduction of material in Chapter 2 that was first published in *Sites: A Journal of Social Anthropology and Cultural Studies.*

1 Introduction to *A Research Agenda for COVID-19 and Society*

Steve Matthewman

COVID-19's impacts are felt at all scales, from micron to the world itself. The pandemic seemingly marks all activities, from intimate interpersonal relations (no more kissing or hand shaking) to global commerce (including unprecedented interruptions to international trade). People have been redeployed as essential workers, found themselves suddenly working from home, been furloughed or made permanently unemployed. Parents have become their children's primary teachers. Shopping – like much work, education and entertainment – is also now increasingly online. Lockdowns have altered our sense of our place in the world and our relationship to others. Multiple boundaries have blurred, including the distinction between physical space and digital space, between home and work, between leisure time and professional time, between economy and society (it turns out that a highly interventionist state is a possibility even in a neoliberal era) and sometimes between individual days as well. As someone put it, every day is 'Blursday'.

Various commentators have noted the novelty of our situation. 'A pandemic such as Covid-19 was widely predicted', wrote Ziauddin Sardar (2021, p. 19):

> But no one imagined that a virus, that most biologists do not even consider as a viable form of life, would stop the twenty-first century, high technology, world in its tracks: stop travel, stop physical contact, stop economic activities, stop growth, stop progress – indeed, stop time itself. Covid-19 demonstrated that it is only when we find ourselves in an unthought future, that we are forced to confront its full implication.

Or, as one of the contributors to this collection (McDonagh) puts it: 'The COVID-19 pandemic has turbocharged world history while ravaging global populations. From digital transformations of work and education, to the development, clinical testing and distribution of new vaccines in unprecedented timeframes, adapting to the virus has driven structural shifts at breakneck speed viewed historically'. Has history stopped or accelerated? It rather depends upon what one is looking at. But at the very least we can agree that the COVID-19 pandemic is historic.

Confronted by this frightening and disorienting reality and the need to understand it, COVID-19 is much discussed, but only partly understood. This volume is designed to add to our comprehension. Like other threatening viruses before it, COVID-19 has precipitated an 'epidemic of signification' (Treichler, 1987). Amongst the weightier meanings generated, COVID-19 is taken to be a signifier of end times, a punishment from God (Dein et al., 2020), a portal between this world and the next (Roy, 2020), an opportunity for international medical cooperation (Buss & Tobar, 2020), an opportunity for fascism to flourish (Davis, 2020, p. 44) and an opportunity for communism to flourish (Žižek, 2020).

The primary vehicle through which the pandemic is apprehended is our language, that core component of consciousness and communication, and consequently of how we think and connect. Quotidian conversation adopted public health discourse. People spoke of bubbles, contact tracing, deep cleans, flattening the curve, achieving herd immunity, lockdown, long haulers, PPE, the R number, self-isolation, social distancing and super-spreaders. New words were coined to describe social practices within our new reality: anti-maskers, the 'rona, coronaskeptics, covidiots, covidivorces, coronapocalypse, doom-scrollers, essential workers, the infodemic, quarintinis, WFH (working from home) and Zoom (Roig–Marín, 2020). The latter becoming 'the default modality for remote engagement, rapidly morphing from brand name to eponymous generic—a verb and a place and mode of being all at once' (Architexturez Research, 2021). Fashion, itself a mode of symbolic communication, has also responded to COVID-19 with dress styles expressing anxiety, frustration and resistance. Hatewear encompasses ensembles that are constantly worn in lockdown despite being neither stylish nor comfortable, while sadwear celebrates clothing that is worn to lift lockdown spirits (Elan, 2021).

Doubtless lives will be parsed into pre-COVID-19 and post-pandemic times. Unique in spatial and temporal terms, this virus affects all people. COVID-19 is everywhere at the same time, and – due to global news networks, ubiquitous social media and near real-time tallies of fatality rates courtesy of advances in digital epidemiology (Ritchie et al., 2021) – *we know it*. Many of the world's remotest regions have also been hit, with infections recorded in Greenland, Montserrat, Rapanui (Easter Island) and even Antarctica (Letzing, 2020; Radio New Zealand, 2020). As of March 2020, three quarters of the world's population were living in countries with stay-at-home commands, over 90 per cent were residing in countries where schools had closed and workplace shutdowns applied in nations responsible for 99 per cent of the planet's Gross Domestic Product (Chossière et al., 2021).

*   *   *

In this collection we offer social science takes on the pandemic and insights into what a research agenda for COVID-19 and society looks like from different disciplinary perspectives. We do not attempt to offer a single party line: people, social arrangements and the pandemic's impacts are far too variegated and complex for that. Instead, we have sought to provide as broad a range as possible from a limited number of contributors. There is a significant disciplinary spread, with authors drawn from: anthropology (Trnka; Wynn), communications (Goode), disaster studies (Dittmer; Lorenz), economics (McDonagh), epidemiology (Wallace & Wallace), Indigenous studies (Lambert), philosophy (Dare; Kingsbury) and sociology (Clark; Craig; Huppatz; Lupton; Matthewman; Southerton; Watson; Wyver). There is also a career spread, with the collection's contributors ranging from early career researchers to emeritus professors. The combined wisdom in these pages is significant. Collectively, they have been publishing from the mid-1970s up to the present day. Those contributors are located in: Australia, Canada, Germany, New Zealand and the United States of America. While much of the discussion has global relevance (Dittmer; Lorenz; Matthewman; Wallace & Wallace), there is a particular focus on Australia (Clark; Craig; Huppatz; Lupton; Southerton; Watson; Wynn), Canada (Lambert), China (McDonagh), New Zealand (Dare; Kingsbury; Trnka), Sweden (Wyver) and the United States (McDonagh), plus a place none of us have yet been to but all of us have an interest in: the future (Goode). The theoretical spread of the work that follows includes: critical disaster studies (Dittmer & Lorenz; Lambert; Matthewman), critical futures studies (Goode), critical whiteness studies (Wyver), evolutionary political economy (McDonagh), phenomenology (Wynn & Trnka) and vital materialism (Southerton, Clark, Watson & Lupton). And various methods are drawn upon in the process, such as: qualitative interviews (Wynn & Trnka), auto-ethnography and ethnography (Wynn & Trnka), case studies (Southerton, Clark, Watson and Lupton) and digital research methods – including digital photo diaries, online interviews and surveys, and video ethnographies (Southerton, Clark, Watson & Lupton; Wynn & Trnka).

Although the disciplinary frames, theories, methods and focus of the respective chapters may differ, there are many commonalities. The pandemic is discussed as a profound social problem throughout. There is the threat of the virus itself, the magnification of already existing inequalities (for example, care burdens and workloads of women, massive asset gains for the wealthy), the stereotyping of some groups (Asians accused of creating it, immigrants and asylum seekers blamed for spreading it). In addition to the pandemic rightly being seen as a problem, there are senses in which social science research into it also presents opportunities. Questions addressed in this collection include: how do we prevent these happening in the future, how do we change the world for the better and how do we do our own work differently?

References

Architexturez Research. (2021). Zoom. *M/C Journal* – Special Issue. 18 March. https://architexturez.net/pst/az-cf-218864-1615558490

Buss, P.M. & Tobar, S. (2020). COVID-19 and Opportunities for International Cooperation in Health. *Cadernos de Saúde Pública* 36(4). https://doi.org/10.1590/0102-311X00066920

Chossière, G. et al. (2021). Air Pollution Impacts of COVID-19–Related Containment Measures. *Science Advances*, 21 May, 7(21). DOI: 10.1126/sciadv.abe1178

Davis, M. (2020). *The Monster Enters: Covid-19, Avian Flu, and the Plagues of Capitalism*. OR Books.

Dein, S. et al. (2020). COVID-19, Mental Health and Religion: An Agenda for Future Research. *Mental Health, Religion & Culture* 23(1), 1–9. DOI:10.1080/13674676.2020.1768725

Elan, P. (2021). 'Hate-wear' and 'Sadwear': Fashion's New Names for Lockdown Dressing. *The Guardian*, 17 January. https://www.theguardian.com/fashion/2021/jan/17/hate-wear-and-sadwear-fashion-new-names-for-covid-lockdown-dressing

Letzing, J. (2020). How Have the Remotest Places on Earth Fared During COVID-19? *World Economic Forum*, 16 July. https://www.weforum.org/agenda/2020/07/how-have-the-remotest-places-on-earth-fared-during-covid-19/

Radio New Zealand. (2020). Covid-19 Cases Recorded in Antarctica at Chilean Research Station. 22 December. https://www.rnz.co.nz/news/world/433435/covid-19-cases-recorded-in-antarctica-at-chilean-research-station

Ritchie, H. et al. (2021). Coronavirus (COVID-19) Deaths. *Our World in Data*. https://ourworldindata.org/coronavirus

Roig–Marín, A. (2020). English-based Coroneologisms: A Short Survey of Our Covid-19-Related Vocabulary. *English Today*, 1–3. doi:10.1017/S0266078420000255

Roy, A. (2020). The Pandemic Is a Portal. *Financial Times*, 4 April. https://www.ft.com/content/10d8f5e8-74eb-11ea-95fe-fcd274e920ca

Sardar, Z. (2021). On the Nature of Time in Postnormal Times. *Journal of Futures Studies* 25(4), 17–30.

Treichler, P.A. (1987). AIDS, Homophobia, and Biomedical Discourse: An Epidemic of Signification. *October 43*(Winter), 31–70. https://doi.org/10.2307/3397564

Žižek, S. (2020). *Pandemic! Covid-19 Shakes the World*. OR Books.

2   COVID-19 and the social sciences

Steve Matthewman

Introduction

While the world has known other pandemics, this one has produced something unprecedented. As the first genuinely global disease, it has ushered in a whole 'new understanding of the vulnerability of the human species qua species' (Arias-Maldonado, 2020).[1] 'One of the first striking features of the pandemic is its planetarity, its contemporaneous and inter-communicated experience on all continents', Göran Therborn (2020) stated. 'Never before in its history has humankind had such a long consciously common experience of life and death'. Thus, unlike previous pandemics, which were analysed retrospectively, and were therefore the domain of history, this pandemic can be analysed in the present, making it fully amenable to the scrutiny of social scientists.

In the material that follows, the resurgence of the social is noted and, by extension, of the social sciences too. The general reasons why disasters lead to an increase in sociality are discussed and the specific ways in which this pandemic has done so. Particular attention is paid to the roles social scientists can play in the context of this pandemic: speaking truth to power, calling out lies and sectional advantage, separating fact from opinion, noting the consequences of political action, predicting social futures (*saying how the world will be*), assessing public opinion (*saying how people would like it to be*), advocating for social justice (*saying how the world should be*) and identifying the mechanisms through which another world can be made possible.

The return of the social

As social scientists we know that we are social beings, that the self is a social construct, that we are enmeshed in networks of mutual dependency, that as a species we rely on social labour to survive. The social is within us (in language, norms, values) as well as beyond us. And we know that, without social contact, we struggle, even die. Indeed, loneliness is now recognised as a significant public health problem. COVID-19 has given the world an object lesson in social science – illuminating the 'constructedness' of society, the radical re-setting of priorities, the possibility of transformational change – such that we can speak of a renewed salience of the social.[2]

Lockdowns showed people the world that we lost. We have had to forego the social contacts, exchanges and rituals that we cherish. Friendships, collegiality and collaboration have all become far more difficult to perform. In this newly sequestered world, we realise 'that the most intimate subject, the most individual and singular, is a social subject' (Dubet, 2021, p. 4). Our sequestration reiterated our dependencies on others, particularly those essential workers provisioning healthcare, food and education. It told us that society is only possible because of the division of labour. It also taught us that some of the less prestigious occupations are also the most important. In addition to reminding us that we all must rely on others, it also reminded us of our reliance upon *systems* (such as those that disburse emergency welfare provisions) and *institutions* (like hospitals). 'With the lockdown, each of us discovers the value of social life' (Dubet, 2021, p. 4).

Physical distancing to prevent contagion is one means through which we demonstrate this, for our individual actions to this end are also generous other-directed acts. It is individuals behaving altruistically for the collective good, putting social welfare above personal desires. (And given the national lockdowns, it was also the privileging of public wellbeing over private profit.) 'Everyone needs everyone to stop the spread, to stop moving, to stop being governed by illusion and delusion, to stop social indulgence and denial', Wendy Brown (2020) wrote. 'Stillness and containment are not individual self-protection but a worldwide mutual social pact'.

Indeed, we have seen the rise of people power the world over responding to COVID-19. Grass roots organisation can be an awesome force. For Garrett M. Graff (2020) '[t]he public's response to the coronavirus will stand as a remarkable moment of national [US] mobilization'. In March 2020, in order to cope with the pandemic, the British government called for a quarter of a million volunteers to come forward to assist senior citizens, those in isolation and frontline medical staff who required supplies delivered. Over three times that amount offered assistance (Solnit, 2020). As George Monbiot chronicles, we have witnessed such acts the world over, from the young volunteers in Hyderabad who are provisioning the city's precarious workers with food packages, to the helpers in Wuhan who are ferrying essential medical workers between hospital and home, to the programmers in Latvia who organised a hackathon to create optimal face shield components for 3D printers, to the student babysitting service in Prague and those groups internationally who are picking up medical supplies for the elderly. 'The shift is even more interesting than it first appears', Monbiot (2020) states. 'Power has migrated not just from private money to the state, but from both market and state to another place altogether: the commons. All over the world, communities have mobilised where governments have failed'.

This 'superbloom of altruistic engagement' (Solnit, 2020) should not surprise. The strengthening of social bonds during times of disaster has been long observed by social scientists. Numerous studies across a century have come to the conclusion that 'disasters bring out prosocial and innovative behaviors in communities' (Knowles, 2011, p.213). Because this phenomenon has been 'discovered' so frequently, it is known by numerous terms within the literature. Common phrases include: 'the brotherhood of pain', 'communitas', 'emergency togetherness', 'extraordinary community', 'post-disaster solidarity', 'post-disaster utopia', 'pro-social behavior', 'social utopia' and 'therapeutic community' (Matthewman & Uekusa, 2021).

Disaster scholars note five reasons for this heightened sociality (see also the chapters by Lambert and Dittmer & Lorenz in this volume). First, it arises because disasters are social phenomena. Threats and damage are public and collectively experienced. Shared risk and suffering bonds survivors. Second, collective action is fostered as current power structures are nowhere near as robust as is commonly thought. They often dissipate or disappoint. Mutual aid from within this 'society of equals' may be the only resource available (Haney, 2018, p.106). Third, this pronounced sense of agency is seen as a vital sense-making activity which yields both affective and applied benefits. Adjustment to the 'new normal' is a coping strategy which enhances both individual and collective wellbeing. Fourth, another major driver for collective action comes from the realisation that disasters (at least those triggered by natural hazards) are often experienced as 'uncontrollable'. No one can be blamed or, if they can, those persons, groups and organisations reside beyond the community. Instead of internal scapegoating and community division, there is a sense of togetherness, a 'democracy of common disaster' (Wood quoted in Kutak, 1938, p.72). Finally, undergirding all of this is the fact that we are essentially social beings. We cannot exist alone. We are products of culture and collective labour. We exist within networks of mutual dependency. We share norms and relations and, to a degree unknown in any other life form, we are remarkably altruistic. As such, we are disposed to assist others (Peek, 2020). Disasters throw this aspect of our species into the sharpest relief.

The connections between personal troubles and public issues have never been clearer. Concepts like the social, the global, figurations and questions like our relationship to authority, the nature of punishment and conformity, the basis of trust – which are so often discussed at a high level of abstraction within the academy – are now viscerally embodied in everyday life. 'The stuff of the tutorial room has become the talk of the town' writes psychology professor Stephen Reicher (2021).

Speaking truth to power

… coronavirus. That sounds like a beautiful place in Italy, right? (President Donald Trump, Campaign Rally in Jacksonville, Florida, 24 September 2020)

There may be senses in which we are all social scientists now. We all have a heightened appreciation of the social, and all of us must have a certain sense of how the world works in order to be competent in it. But social scientists claim that their knowledge is more robust and reliable than the wisdom of common sense. This is particularly important given concerns about the 'infodemic', the prevalence of false and misleading health information, often propagated through social media networks (World Health Organization, 2021).

Zygmunt Bauman and Tim May (2019, pp. 4–10) note that social science (they were specifically writing about sociology) is superior to common sense in key ways:

1. The commitment to responsible speech (discussed below)
2. The size of the field – it moves beyond an individualistic frame to consider the experiences of multiple life worlds
3. The way it makes sense of human reality by situating agency and personal interactions within the context of the social forces, institutional structures, network effects and interdependencies that make our lives what they are
4. By applying strategies of 'defamiliarisation' which unsettles what is taken for granted, subjecting everything to critical scrutiny

Let us elaborate the point about responsible speech. This is part of sociology's scientific ethos. In the common-sense scheme of things, you can say whatever you like. By contrast, sociologists – and social scientists more generally – are careful to distinguish fact from value and tested findings from beliefs. There is a vigilance to social science thinking as well as clarity and transparency in this process. Social scientists must show their reasoning and present their evidence (unlike certain political leaders we cannot become post-truth or peddle alternative facts). They should be open to scrutiny and they should consider the veracity of alternative viewpoints and propositions.

Part of that commitment to responsible speech also entails speaking truth to power. The powerful have the ability to broker our reality, to successfully name and classify the world, to say what can exist and how the world should be. They have the ability to determine the horizons of our existence, stipulating what is acceptable, what is thinkable and what is possible, what can be said and done (Bourdieu, 2018). Such actions may be in their own sectional interest rather than for the greater public good. Social scientists should openly state when this is the case.

There are additional reasons for social science intervention here: the powerful need to be held to account as they lie. As evidence of this one need look no further than the then-world's most powerful man: President Donald Trump. On 2 March 2020 he said: 'My administration has also taken the most aggressive action in modern history to protect Americans from the coronavirus'. Social science fact checkers have made a mockery of this claim. And this was but one of Trump's falsehoods about COVID-19. Other lies and poor advice in the first nine months of 2020 included: questioning the efficacy of masks; promoting false cures such as convalescent plasma, disinfectant, hydroxychloroquine and ultraviolet rays; undermining his own health officials, notably Dr Fauci but also the Centers for Disease Control and Prevention; falsely claiming to have the virus 'under control' very early in the pandemic; racialising the virus (even referring to it as 'Kung Flu' and the 'Chinese virus'); spuriously claiming that COVID-19 would go away as temperatures rose; urging governors to open their states well in advance of any vaccine rollout; suggesting shutdowns are more problematic than the virus itself; stating that large gatherings of unvaccinated crowds are 'very safe'; saying that testing is 'overrated'; noting that without testing there would be 'no cases'; arguing that only the elderly with pre-existing conditions are vulnerable to COVID-19; consistently saying that the virus would just go away; and routinely lying about rates of infection and death in the United States while over-inflating excess mortality rates in Europe (Kiely et al., 2020).

Similarly, on the other side of the Atlantic, one of Prime Minister Boris Johnson's very first press conferences began: 'I must level with the British public: many more families are going to lose loved ones before their time' (quoted in Stewart et al., 2020). Instead of implementing widespread testing, tracking and tracing and enforcing social distancing and outright lockdown to flatten the curve, they opted for herd immunity, which is an ill-advised strategy absent an effective vaccine. Isabel Frey notes how this logic aligns with neoliberal ideology: it belies the people-before-profits tenet of the country's economics, and the state's relinquishment of responsibility in this privatised environment (for more on the topic of herd immunity see Wyver's chapter; and for additional critiques of neoliberalism see Wallace & Wallace, 2016). If you are at risk, poor, precarious or unemployed, it is your own fault for not competing adequately in the market. For her, herd immunity is nothing other than 'epidemiological neoliberalism', a strategy of letting the epidemic, much like the market, go unregulated (Frey, 2020). Speaking truth to power here means calling them out for their erroneous approach and noting its consequences. It also emerges that pitting the economy against public health is an entirely false binary. Here, then, is another role for the social scientist: the debunker of myths. Research has shown that the United Kingdom would have saved 65 000 lives had it adopted a very strict style of lockdown early on and its Gross Domestic Product would only have fallen 0.5 per cent instead of the 11 per cent that it did (Aum et al., 2021).

It's the end of the world as we know it? Prognostication and its perils

The desire to predict events is one of the rationales for all of the social sciences (Hechter, 1995, p. 1520), and the ability to accurately do so within a field shows that a scientific endeavour has reached maturity (Kaplan, 1940, p. 492). Within the academy and beyond, prognostic skills are also a basis for claiming relevance. We have no shortage of predictions when it comes to COVID-19.

Albena Azmanova (2020) argues that pandemic responses have marked a radical disjuncture with the old normal in three key ways. First, lockdowns around the globe have shown that serving the economy is not the sine qua non of government. Contra neoliberal orthodoxy, private profit does not have to take precedence over everything else. Second, the inability of even the wealthiest countries to secure public wellbeing shows that those societies are also afflicted by a widespread pathogen – that of precarity. As a result, elites have lost their legitimacy. They have been shown to govern in the interests of themselves alone, and all too often democracy has given way to authoritarianism. Third, the virus has disproportionately impacted the most marginalised communities. Pre-pandemic their precarity may have rendered them servile. But in exposing the false promises of neoliberalism and by magnifying already-existing injustices, oppressed groups will be galvanised into action. One manifestation of this is the 'Great Resignation', as workers have voluntarily resigned en masse, a counterintuitive phenomenon in a time of economic downturn. But COVID-19 has shown the emptiness of many of neoliberalism's promises and forced people to reassess their own life priorities (Kaplan, 2021).

For Bob de Wit (2021), this coronavirus will catalyse a social revolution, ushering in 'Society 4.0'. In his four-stage schema, the first society to emerge was an agrarian one. Settled agriculture displaced hunter–gatherers. The second society saw a shift from agriculture to trade and the onset of economic globalisation. The third social formation of note was driven by industrialisation, inaugurating mechanised labour. Now we must reckon with its negative consequences. In so doing, we must usher in Society 4.0 in order to replace extractive industries with regenerative ones.

Azmanova and de Wit are amongst a group of scholars predicting that the pandemic will be an 'event' in the Foucauldian sense (Foucault, 1984), which is to say it will be a genuine break in history, leading to new forms of social arrangements. Slavoj Žižek (2020) concurs: 'It's time to accept that the pandemic has changed the way we exist forever. Now the human race has to embark on the profoundly difficult and painful process of deciding what form the 'new normality' is going to take'. The UN's Health Chief, Tedros Adhanom Ghebreyesus, thought much the same: 'we will not be going back to the "old normal"'. The pandemic has already changed the way we live our lives. Part of adjusting to the 'new normal' is finding ways to live our lives safely' (UN News, 2020). The broader commentariat have also announced that COVID-19 has ended the world as we knew it. A partial list of such pronouncements includes the end of asylum (Ghezelbash, 2020), cash (Barrigan, 2020), cars and commuting (Anon, 2020; Fengler, 2020), big cities (Tavernise & Mervosh, 2020), mass protests (Brannen, 2020), democracy (Repucci & Slipowitz, 2020), globalisation (Gray, 2020), US hegemony (Norrlöf, 2020), neoliberalism (Saad-Filho, 2020) and capitalism (Mason, 2020).

Historians can lend some credence to claims of imminent – and significant – transformation. Walter Scheidel (2017) notes that there are only four major phenomena that have made for a more equal society: war, revolution, state failure and pandemic. He argues that pandemics have had the greatest impact. The most spectacular example of this comes from the worst plague of them all: The Black Death. This pandemic killed a third of the world's population. The horrors of this plague are well known. The collective consequences and responses less so. Survivors could find no divine purpose in it. The power of Church and nobility were challenged. The workings of God and the idea of a fixed feudal order were sharply questioned. 'To that extent the Black Death may have been the unrecognized beginning of modern man' (Tuchman, 1978,

p. 123). Across Europe and beyond, agricultural workers and craftspersons leveraged the chronic labour shortages to agitate for better pay and conditions. Working hours shortened while wages increased. Most doubled, some tripled (Pamuk, 2007).

Yet social scientists should be mindful of the perils of punditry. The Global Health Security Index (2019) ranked the United States of America and the United Kingdom first and second in terms of their ability to counter large-scale infectious disease outbreaks. COVID-19 made a mockery of this prediction, as both countries struggled to implement widespread testing, to provision frontline healthcare workers with sufficient personal protective equipment or to secure adequate numbers of hospital beds. Authorities in these countries failed to contain the disease or even predict a single parameter of COVID-19. An article published in *The Lancet* castigated both national governments for being about as far from best practice as it is possible to be. The outright lies and mismanagement of the former and the quasi-criminal delays of the latter 'have provided among the world's worst responses to the pandemic', Sarah Dalglish (2020, p. 1189) observed. As of late February 2021, the United States passed a grim milestone. Half a million people had died of COVID-19 in that country, accounting for a fifth of the world's fatalities. This figure approximates the American war dead from World War Two, Korea and Vietnam combined (Hollingsworth & Webber, 2021). At the time of writing, the United States has recorded the most COVID-19 deaths globally. The United Kingdom has the third worst overall death rate in the world.

This is but one of many examples showing the failures of prediction and the shortcomings of expertise. As such, we would do well to heed Andy Sterling's (2020) warnings: 'For whatever happens next, what is already evident is that: expert advisers and scientific institutions found themselves so wrong; commentators and policy-makers so short-sighted; affluent societies so poorly resourced; macho demagogues and plutocrats so indecisive; and democracies and autocracies alike so ill-prepared'. Amongst the many potential casualties of the pandemic – just-in-time production systems, neoliberalism, even capitalism itself – perhaps the only one we should actually seek to endorse is the pretence to predictive control (Sterling, 2020; and see the closing chapter by Goode on post-pandemic futures).

Utopia or bust: demanding the impossible

The future is hard to predict and impossible to control, but this does not mean that we should cease our efforts to make the world a better place. Albion Small said that sociology was 'born of the modern zeal to make society better' (quoted in Bauman, 2011, p. 160). This social justice impulse is to be found across the social sciences.

For sociologists, utopia is more than just an idea; it is also a method. Ruth Levitas (2013, p. 153) identifies three sociological approaches to utopia as method. The first she calls an archaeological mode – extracting ideas of the good society from political doctrines, and social and economic policies. The second is ontological – looking at what types of people societies promote and enable. In other words, what types of human flourishing are (and are not) permitted within the prevailing social structures. The third mode is architectural – imagining better future worlds, and what they may be like for those who would live in them.

Progressive change may appear impossible. It will be presented as such by those with the most to gain from the current social order. The powerful typically oppose change as they profit most from the status quo. It is in their interests to disseminate ideologies that cement current social arrangements, and that make them appear natural rather than constructed. It is for this reason that Mark Fisher (2009, p. 18) stated that 'emancipatory politics must always destroy the appearance of a "natural order", must reveal what is presented as necessary and inevitable to be a mere contingency, just as it must make what was previously deemed to be impossible seem attainable'.

As German sociologist Sebastian Scheerer (1986, p. 7) wrote, 'there has never been a major social transformation in the history of mankind that had not been looked upon as unrealistic, idiotic, or utopian by the large majority of experts even a few years before the unthinkable became reality'. Amongst such 'unthinkable' transformations we can list the abolition of slavery, the end of the British Empire, the collapse of the Soviet Union and the culmination of the Cold War, the rise of animal rights and, more recently, the embrace of marriage equality in various parts of the world. For all of these reasons we should revive the slogan of the student revolts of 1968: 'Be realistic – demand the impossible'. Such struggles are worth our while. As Hannah Arendt said of the fight for women's liberation: 'The real question to ask is, what will we lose if we win?' (quoted in Honig, 2009, p. 66).

The seemingly 'impossible' has already happened. The lockdown showed that a supposedly unstoppable global economic system that should be privileged above all else – *There is No Alternative* – can actually be forced to a halt. 'The pandemic has shown us the economy is a very narrow and limited way of organising life and deciding who is important and who is not important', offered Bruno Latour (2020). In demonstrating that capitalism can yield to public wellbeing, the lockdown also provided a time of contemplation, a moment to consider individual and collective futures, what we might need and what we might want, to think about the elements of our pre-COVID-19 existence that should be retained and what should be jettisoned. Moreover, it has also made it clear that ideas and knowledge can be transferred as easily as viruses.

Other 'impossibilities' were soon realised: homelessness was ended in Aotearoa New Zealand (Davidson, 2020), free childcare was provided in Australia (Department of Education, Skills and Employment, 2020), hospitals have been nationalised in Spain and private hospitals taken over in Ireland (Payne, 2020; Mercille et al., 2021), basic income has been granted in Canada (BBC, 2020), migrants and asylum seekers have been given full citizenship in Portugal (Schengenvisainfo News, 2020) and Spain has launched a trial of a four-day working week (Kassam, 2021).

COVID-19 has shown that social structures can change quite rapidly. Social science research also shows that progressive changes are desired. Most Britons who were surveyed in a YouGov poll hoped that they personally, and their country generally, would change for the better following the pandemic. A mere nine per cent of those questioned wanted to return to the status quo ante (Binding, 2020). A Kudos Organisational Dynamics survey of 1000 people found that 81 per cent of respondents thought that the coronavirus pandemic will leave behind a society that has learned good lessons about 'being in it together and being kind', and 88 per cent of those surveyed believed that this sense of community would either continue or grow post-lockdown (Lourens, 2020, pp. 2–3). A Massey University study showed that seven out of ten New Zealanders wanted a green COVID-19 recovery. The majority of those questioned said they were going to change to more environmentally friendly practices in the next year even if it inconvenienced them and cost them more (Morton, 2020). One of the most comprehensive surveys to date was produced by IPSOS. They gathered the opinions of 21 000 adults in 27 countries in work undertaken on behalf of the World Economic Forum. The results showed that almost 90 per cent of respondents wanted a fairer world post–COVID-19. And of those questioned, almost three quarters – 72 per cent – would like their life to change markedly rather than have it return to the pre-COVID-19 normal. Moreover, 86 per cent would like to see *significant* positive transformation in the world, particularly in terms of social and environmental justice (IPSOS, 2020).

Conclusion

This chapter has addressed the magnitude of COVID-19's impacts and the role of social science in assessing them. The argument has been made that COVID-19 has forced appreciation of, and focus on, the social. With this comes renewed relevance for the social sciences. Indeed, for Stephen Reicher (2021), 'COVID has more effectively demonstrated the importance of the social sciences to a sceptical public and a dismissive government than years of campaigning'. The pandemic has shown us that another world is possible. Confronted by rapid change, crisis and a desire for better alternatives, social scientists can guide actions. For as Walby (2021, p.25) notes, 'a theory of society is needed' (and see Dubet, 2021, p.4). Not only is another world possible, social science research shows that another world is desired. The overwhelming majority of those surveyed would like to live in ways that are far more equitable and sustainable. This necessitates the utilisation of utopia as method: identifying notions of the good society, fostering human flourishing and imagining a better world than this one.

Social scientists have garnered numerous solutions to these ends, with two of our biggest challenges in mind: unprecedented wealth disparities and unparalleled environmental threats. On the former, guaranteed jobs in the public service or voluntary sector funded by government (Tcherneva, 2020) would pull a lot of products, activities and services out of the market and help to redefine collective needs and desires. This could be supplemented by expanded welfare provisions – including such things as free health and education, basic income, progressive taxation, a public banking service based on central bank digital currencies and the redistribution of inheritance. Piketty (2021) suggests that everyone receive a minimum inheritance at 25 since concentration of property is one of inequality's biggest drivers. In France he sets this at 60 per cent of the average wealth per adult, suggesting it be paid from progressive taxation and wealth taxes.

It would make sense to set these new policies within the broader context of a Green New Deal. Amongst other things this seeks to attain net-zero greenhouse gas emissions, secure clean air and water, climate and community resilience and a sustainable environment for all. As Ann Pettifor (2019) notes, the overriding aim is for a steady state or circular economy. It should not exceed ecological limits (for example atmospheric aerosol loading). It should look to minimise waste and maximise recycling. There should be less focus on frivolous consumption, more focus on local production and cooperation, and a just transition to renewable energies.

Writing in *Climate & Capitalism*, Andreas Malm (2018) suggests a ten-point programme, beginning with a moratorium on all new facilities for extracting fossil fuels. He also advocates for the shift to 100 per cent renewable energy, and he calls for an end to the expansion of air, sea and road travel (with existing road and sea travel converted to electricity and wind power). Mass transit systems should be expanded – and scaled up where possible. Local food supplies should replace airfreighted goods. Massive reforestation programmes should commence. Old buildings should be insulated; new ones should generate their own zero-carbon power. Plant proteins should replace the global meat industry. Public investment should be geared towards sustainable renewable energy technologies and those capable of carbon sequestration.

The material above deals with production of inequality, which is important, because suffering tends to fracture along the familiar fault lines of age, gender, ethnicity and social class (another skill that social scientists possess is that of pattern recognition). Work by disaster scholars reveals remarkably consistent patterns in which the isolated, weak and less wealthy consistently fare worse (Matthewman, 2015, pp. 13, 20). Infection fatality rate (IFR) is correlated with age. The elderly are feeling coronavirus' physical impacts the most. In terms of social impacts, it could be that the youth are most affected by the lockdown. They are having to forgo work and their education is being compromised. The pandemic is racialised. Asians are being scapegoated and attacked for spreading the virus (Tavernise & Oppel Jr, 2020), while official statistics show marked differences between black and white IFRs (Timothy, 2020). Indigenous groups are also at great risk. In Aotearoa New Zealand the 'estimated IFR for Māori is around 50% higher than non-Māori' (Steyn et al., 2020; and see Lambert in this collection). There is an obvious gender component too. Women are on the frontline of coronavirus. The majority of the planet's healthcare and social care workers are female. The World Health Organization (WHO) puts the figure at 70 per cent (Boniol et al., 2019). And this statistic only considers paid care. Women appear more likely to lose their jobs because of COVID-19, and they are more prone to domestic violence because of its many stressors, such that it has been referred to as the 'shadow pandemic' (UN Women, 2021; and see the chapter by Huppatz & Craig). Paula Braverman (2020) made the point cogently when she wrote for the UNESCO Inclusive Policy Lab: 'Inequality is our pre-existing condition'.

Having dealt with the production of inequality, we must also deal with the production of pandemics. As Larry Brilliant, one of the WHO figures central to the eradication of smallpox, said: 'Outbreaks are inevitable. Pandemics are optional' (quoted in Matthewman, 2015, p. 27). The independent scientific task force Preventing Pandemics at the Source (2021) has identified the root cause of pandemics over the last century as human-driven viral spillover. In particular, they call for an end to practices of deforestation and forest fragmentation, and of commercial wildlife trade and markets. They would also like to see improved farm biosecurity. Yet we also need to reckon with global capitalist agribusiness because their reconfiguration of landscapes and ecosystems has proven to be profitable for more than multinational capital (see the following chapter by Wallace & Wallace). A host of infectious diseases that similarly prey upon people have benefitted from deforestation and plantation monocultures. In the first instance, forest depletion removes the barrier between humans and viruses that are endemic to avian and animal populations. Corporate agriculture's intense production cycles undermine ecosystem resilience and fast-track pathogen transfer. Global commodity chains ensure that bacteria and viruses from the most isolated hinterlands can enter the very heart of our most densely populated cities. The 2013 Ebola outbreak in West Africa was a paradigmatic example of a pandemic created by this very constellation of factors (Wallace and Wallace, 2016). Rob Wallace (2017) sees the end of corporate capitalist agriculture as being the only way to truly eradicate the pandemic problem. Local farmers and local communities must be in control of their own lands. 'Public trusts and cooperative models organized around multifunctional agroecologies addressing the needs of food and farmer and environment all together are our best protection against the worst of the new diseases'.

Social science research consistently shows that prevention is cheaper than cure. Every dollar spent on mitigation usually saves spending up to thirteen times that amount on post-disaster recovery (Multihazard Mitigation Council cited in FEMA, 2008; National Institute of Building Sciences, 2020). In the case of pandemics, the return on investment is far more favourable. Spending money on prevention could be more than 100 times cheaper than dealing with their deadly consequences (Harrabin, 2020). Given all of the above, social science work is needed now more than ever.

Notes

1   One could surmise that unprecedented wealth disparities, entry into the Age of the Anthropocene and the prospect of the sixth mass extinction event also add to the zeitgeist.

2   For example, a tweet by Mohamad Safa made the front page of *Reddit* on 2 February 2021. It had over 100 000 views. It read: 'What we learned in 2020? That oil is worthless in a society without consumption. That healthcare has to be public because health is public. That 50% of jobs can be done from home while the other 50% deserve more than they're being paid. That we live in a society, not an economy'. A tweet sent by blondie wasabi on 14 March 2020 had garnered 282 000 likes. It read: 'it's crazy how because of corona we can see how almost everything we do is a totally made up social construct that can be instantly stopped if we wanted to lol'.

References

Anon. (2020). The End of Commuterland. *The Economist*, 12 September: 21–22.

Arias-Maldonado, M. (2020). COVID-19 as a Global Risk: Confronting the Ambivalences of a Socionatural Threat. *Societies 10*(4): 92. DOI:10.3390/soc10040092

Aum, S., S.Y.L. & Shin, Y. (2021). Inequality of Fear and Self-quarantine: Is There a Trade-off Between GDP and Public Health? *Journal of Public Economics 194*, February. https://doi.org/10.1016/j.jpubeco.2020.104354

Azmanova, A. (2020). Viral Insurgencies: Can Capitalism Survive COVID? *Theory & Event 23*(4): Supplement. https://muse.jhu.edu/article/775405

Barrigan, D. (2020). Will Covid-19 Spell the End for Cash? *Finextra*, 30 September. https://www.finextra.com/blogposting/19378/will-covid-19-spell-the-end-for-cash

Bauman, Z. (2011). *Collateral Damage: Social Inequalities in a Global Age*. Polity Press.

Bauman, Z. & May, T. (2019). *Thinking Sociologically*, 3rd edn. John Wiley & Sons.

BBC. (2020). Canada Backs $75bn Coronavirus Relief Bill. 25 March. https://www.bbc.com/news/world-us-canada-52022506

Binding, L. (2020). Coronavirus: Only 9% of Britons Want Life to Return to 'Normal' Once Lockdown Is Over. *Sky News*, 17 April. https://news.sky.com/story/coronavirus-only-9-of-britons-want-life-to-return-to-normal-once-lockdown-is-over-11974459

Boniol, M., McIsaac, M., Xu, L., Wuliji, T., Diallo, K. & Campbell, J. (2019). FedGender Equity in the Health Workforce: Analysis of 104 Countries. *World Health Organization*. https://apps.who.int/iris/bitstream/handle/10665/311314/WHO-HIS-HWF-Gender-WP1-2019.1-eng.pdf

Bourdieu, P. (2018). *Classification Struggles*. Polity Press.

Brannen, S. (2020). Will COVID-19 End the Age of Mass Protests? *Center for Strategic and International Studies*, 7 April. https://www.csis.org/analysis/will-covid-19-end-age-mass-protests

Braverman, P. (2020). COVID-19: Inequality Is Our Pre-Existing Condition. *UNESCO Inclusive Policy Lab*, 14 April. https://en.unesco.org/inclusivepolicylab/news/covid-19-inequality-our-pre-existing-condition

Brown, W. (2020). From Exposure to Manifestation. *LA Review of Books*, 14 April. https://lareviewofbooks.org/article/quarantine-files-thinkers-self-isolation/#_ftn4

Dalglish, S.L. (2020). COVID-19 Gives the Lie to Global Health Expertise. *The Lancet*, 11 April. DOI:10.1016/S0140-6736(20)30739-X

Davidson, I. (2020). COVID 19 Coronavirus: Rough Sleeping all but Eliminated in New Zealand as Pandemic Crisis Frees up Motels and Housing. *New Zealand Herald*, 22 May. https://www.nzherald.co.nz/nz/news/article.cfm?c_id=1&objectid=12333758

De Wit, B. (2021). *Society 4.0: Resolving Eight Key Issues to Build a Citizens Society*. Vakmedianet.

Department of Education, Skills and Employment. (2020). COVID-19: Early Childhood Education and Care Relief Package. *Australian Government*, 2 April. http://www.earlychildhoodaustralia.org.au/media/eca-covid-19-response/

Dubet, F. (2021). The Return of Society. *European Journal of Social Theory 24*(1): 3–21.

Federal Emergency Management Agency (FEMA). (2008). Mitigation's Value to Society. https://www.fema.gov/pdf/hazard/hurricane/2008/gustav/mitigations_value_factsheet2008.pdf

Fengler, W. (2020). The End of the Car as We Know It: What COVID-19 Means to Mobility in Europe. *Brookings*, 28 September. https://www.brookings.edu

/blog/future-development/2020/09/28/the-end-of-the-car-as-we-know-it-what-covid
-19-means-to-mobility-in-europe/

Fisher, M. (2009). *Capitalist Realism: Is There No Alternative?* John Hunt Publishing.

Foucault, M. (1984). What Is Enlightenment? In P. Rabinow (Ed.) *The Foucault Reader* (pp. 32–50), Pantheon Books.

Frey, I. (2020). 'Herd Immunity' Is Epidemiological Neoliberalism. *The Quarantimes*, 19 March. https://thequarantimes.wordpress.com/2020/03/19/herd-immunity-is
-epidemiological-neoliberalism/

Ghezelbash, D. (2020). COVID-19 and the End of Asylum. Andrew and Renata Kaldor Centre for International Refugee Law, 11 June. https://www.kaldorcentre.unsw.edu
.au/publication/covid-19-and-end-asylum

GHS Index. (2019). The Global Health Security Index. Center for Health Security, Johns Hopkins University. https://www.ghsindex.org/wp-content/uploads/2019
/10/2019-Global-Health-Security-Index.pdf

Graff, G.M. (2020). What Americans Are Doing Now Is Beautiful: The Public's Response to the Coronavirus Will Stand as a Remarkable Moment of National Mobilization. *The Atlantic*, 19 March. https://www.theatlantic.com/ideas/archive/2020/03/inspiring
-galvanizing-beautiful-spirit-2020/608308/

Gray, N.H. (2020). Will COVID-19 Put an End to Globalization? *Scoop*, 16 August. https://www.scoop.co.nz/stories/PO2008/S00199/will-covid-19-put-an-end-to
-globalization.htm

Haney, T.J. (2018). Paradise Found? The Emergence of Social Capital, Place Attachment, and Civic Engagement After Disaster. *International Journal of Mass Emergencies and Disasters 36*(2): 97–119.

Harrabin, R. (2020). Cheaper to Prevent Pandemics Than 'Cure' Them. BBC News, 30 October. https://www.bbc.com/news/science-environment-54721687

Hechter, M. (1995). Introduction: Reflections on Historical Prophecy in the Social Sciences. Symposium on Prediction in the Social Sciences. *American Journal of Sociology 100*(6): 1520–27.

Hollingsworth, H. & Webber, T. (2021). US Tops 500,000 Virus Deaths, Matching the Toll of 3 Wars. *Associated Press*, 23 February. https://apnews.com/article
/us-over-500k-coronavirus-deaths-4ffa86c709f6a843de9cf0711e7215cf

Honig, B. (2009). *Emergency Politics: Paradox, Law, Democracy*. Princeton University Press.

IPSOS. (2020). Around the World, People Yearn for Significant Change Rather Than a Return to a 'Pre-COVID Normal'. 16 September. https://www.ipsos.com/en
/global-survey-unveils-profound-desire-change-rather-return-how-life-and-world
-were-covid-19

Kaplan, J. (2012). The Psychologist Who Coined the Phrase 'Great Resignation' Reveals How He Saw It Coming and Where He Sees It Going. 'Who We Are as an Employee and as a Worker Is Very Central to Who We Are'. *Business Insider*, 2 October. https://www.businessinsider.com.au/why-everyone-is-quitting-great-resignation
-psychologist-pandemic-rethink-life-2021-10

Kaplan, O. (1940). Prediction in the Social Sciences. *Philosophy of Science 7*(4): 492–498.

Kassam, A. (2021). Spain to Launch Trial of Four-day Working Week. *The Guardian*, 15 March. https://www.theguardian.com/world/2021/mar/15/spain-to
-launch-trial-of-four-day-working-week

Kiely, E., Robertson, L., Rieder, R. & Gore, D. (2020). Timeline of Trump's COVID-19 Comments. *FactCheck.org*, 2 October. https://www.factcheck.org/2020/10
/timeline-of-trumps-covid-19-comments/

Knowles, S.G. (2011). *The Disaster Experts: Mastering Risk in Modern America*. University of Pennsylvania Press.

Kutak, R.I. (1938). The Sociology of Crises: The Louisville Flood of 1937. *Social Forces, 17*(1): 66–72.

Latour, B. (2020). This Is a Global Catastrophe That Has Come from Within: Interview with Jonathan Watts. *The Guardian*, 6 June. https://www.theguardian .com/world/2020/jun/06/bruno-latour-coronavirus-gaia-hypothesis-climate -crisis

Levitas, R. (2013). *Utopia as Method*. Palgrave Macmillan.

Lourens, M. (2020). A Snapshot of Lockdown Shows Big Changes. *The Sunday Star-Times*, 19 April: 2–3.

Malm, A. (2018). Revolutionary Strategy in a Warming World. *Climate & Capitalism*, 17 March. https://climateandcapitalism.com/2018/03/17/malm-revolutionary-strategy/

Mason, P. (2020). Will Coronavirus Signal the End of Capitalism? *Aljazeera*, 3 April. https://www.aljazeera.com/opinions/2020/4/3/will-coronavirus-signal-the -end-of-capitalism

Matthewman, S. (2015). *Disasters, Risks and Revelation: Making Sense of Our Times*. Palgrave Macmillan.

Matthewman, S. & Uekusa, S. (2021). Theorizing Disaster Communitas. *Theory & Society 50*: 965–984. https://doi.org/10.1007/s11186-021-09442-4

Mercille, J., Turner, B. & Lucey, D.S. (2021). Ireland's Takeover of Private Hospitals During the COVID-19 Pandemic. *Health Econ Policy Law* (1–6). https://doi :10.1017/S1744133121000189

Monbiot, G. (2020). The Horror Films Got It Wrong. This Virus Has Turned Us into Caring Neighbours. *The Guardian*, 31 March. https://www.theguardian.com /commentisfree/2020/mar/31/virus-neighbours-covid-19

Morton, J. (2020). Seven in 10 Kiwis Want a Green COVID-19 Recovery – Survey. *New Zealand Herald*, 4 August. https://www.nzherald.co.nz/nz/seven -in-10-kiwis-want-a-green-covid-19-recovery-survey/L2A4KL6EWYMLNFHKALO 43LPN54/

National Institute of Building Sciences. (2020). Mitigation Saves: Mitigation Saves up to $13 per $1 Invested. http://2021.nibs.org/files/pdfs/ms_v4_overview.pdf

Norrlöf, C. (2020). Is COVID-19 the End of US Hegemony? Public Bads, Leadership Failures and Monetary Hegemony. *International Affairs 96*(5): 1281–1303. https:// doi.org/10.1093/ia/iiaa134

Pamuk, Ş. (2007). The Black Death and the Origins of the 'Great Divergence' Across Europe, 1300–1600. *European Review of Economic History 11*: 289–317.

Payne, A. (2020). Spain Has Nationalized All of Its Private Hospitals as the Country Goes into Coronavirus Lockdown. *Business Insider*, 17 March. https://www.businessinsider .com.au/coronavirus-spain-nationalises-private-hospitals-emergency-covid-19 -lockdown-2020-3?r=US&IR=T

Peek, L. (2020). The Ties that Bind. *The Natural Hazards Center*, 20 March. https:// hazards.colorado.edu/news/director/the-ties-that-bind

Pettifor, A. (2019). *The Case for the Green New Deal*. Verso.

Piketty, T. (2021). From Basic Income to Inheritance for All. *Le Blog de Thomas Piketty*, 18 May. https://www.lemonde.fr/blog/piketty/category/in-english/

Preventing Pandemics at the Source (2021). Statement released by the Coalition on Preventing Pandemics at the Source in advance of the 74th World Health Assembly, 20 May. https://72d37324-5089-459c-8f70-271d19427cf2.filesusr.com/ugd/056cf4 _ee875107e8164637a9ab42648c5775ec.pdf

Reicher, S. (2021). For Psychologists, the Pandemic Has Shown People's Capacity for Cooperation. *The Guardian*, 2 January. https://www.theguardian.com /commentisfree/2021/jan/02/psychologists-pandemic-cooperation-government-public -britain?CMP=Share_iOSApp_Other

Repucci, S. & Slipowitz, A. (2020). The Impact of COVID-19 on the Global Struggle for Freedom. *Freedom House*. Washington DC. https://freedomhouse.org/report /special-report/2020/democracy-under-lockdown

Saad-Filho, A. (2020). From COVID-19 to the End of Neoliberalism. *Critical Sociology* 46(4–5): 477–485. https://doi.org/10.1177/0896920520929966

Scheidel, W. (2017). *The Great Leveller: Violence and the History of Inequality from the Stone Age to the Twenty-First Century*. Princeton University Press.

Scheerer, S. (1986). Towards Abolitionism. *Contemporary Crises 10*(1): 5–20.

Schengenvisainfo News. (2020). Portugal Grants Migrants and Asylum Seekers Full Citizenship Rights During COVID-19 Outbreak. 2 April. https://www .schengenvisainfo.com/news/portugal-grants-migrants-and-asylum-seekers-full -citizenship-rights-during-covid-19/

Solnit, R. (2020). 'The Way We Get Through This Is Together': The Rise of Mutual Aid Under Coronavirus. *The Guardian*, 14 May. https://www.theguardian.com /world/2020/may/14/mutual-aid-coronavirus-pandemic-rebecca-solnit

Sterling, A. (2020). Modernity Without Its Clothes: The Pandemic Crisis Shines a Light on Futilities of Control. Steps Centre: Pathways to Sustainability. 7 April. https:// steps-centre.org/blog/modernity-without-its-clothes-the-pandemic-crisis-shines-a -light-on-futilities-of-control/

Stewart, H., Proctor, K. & Siddique, H. (2020). Johnson: Many More People Will Lose Loved Ones to Coronavirus. *The Guardian*, 12 March. https://www.theguardian. com/world/2020/mar/12/uk-moves-to-delay-phase-of-coronavirus-plan

Steyn, N. et al. (2020). Estimated Inequities in COVID-19 Infection Fatality Rates by Ethnicity for Aotearoa New Zealand. *Te Pūnaha Matatini*. https://cpb-ap-se2 .wpmucdn.com/blogs.auckland.ac.nz/dist/d/75/files/2020/04/Estimated-ifrs_draft 12.ACTUALFINAL.pdf

Tavernise, S. & Mervosh, S. (2020). America's Biggest Cities Were Already Losing Their Allure. What Happens Next? *New York Times (Online)*, 19 April. https://www .nytimes.com/2020/04/19/us/coronavirus-moving-city-future.html

Tavernise, S. & Oppel, R.A. (2020). Spit On, Yelled At, Attacked: Chinese-Americans Fear for Their Safety. *New York Times*, 23 March. https://www.nytimes.com/2020/03/23 /us/chinese-coronavirus-racist-attacks.html

Tcherneva, P.R. (2020). *The Case for a Job Guarantee*. Polity.

Therborn, G. (2020). Opus Magnum: How the Pandemic Is Changing the World. *Living and Thinking Crisis: Thesis Eleven*, 6 July. https://thesiseleven.com/2020/07/06 /opus-magnum-how-the-pandemic-is-changing-the-world/

Timothy, R.K. (2020). Coronavirus Is Not the Great Equalizer – Race Matters. *The Conversation*, 7 April. https://theconversation.com/coronavirus-is-not-the-great -equalizer-race-matters-133867

Tuchman, B. (1978). *A Distant Mirror: The Calamitous 14th Century*. Ballantine Books.

UN News. (2020). COVID-19: No Return to 'Old Normal', Says UN Health Chief, as Cases Top 15 million. 23 July. https://news.un.org/en/story/2020/07/1068941

UN Women. (2021). The Shadow Pandemic: Violence against Women during COVID-19. https://www.unwomen.org/en/news/in-focus/in-focus-gender-equality-in-covid -19-response/violence-against-women-during-covid-19

Walby, S. (2021). The COVID Pandemic and Social Theory: Social Democracy and Public Health in the Crisis. *European Journal of Social Theory 24*: 22–43. https://doi.org/10.1177/1368431020970127

Wallace, R. (2017). Capitalism and Pathogens: Ten Theses on Farming and Disease. *Climate & Capitalism*, 8 June. https://climateandcapitalism.com/2017/06/08/ten-theses-on-farming-and-disease/

Wallace, R. & Wallace, R. (2016). Ebola's Ecologies: Agro-Economics and Epidemiology in West Africa. *New Left Review 102*: 43–55.

World Health Organization. (2021). Infodemic. https://www.who.int/health-topics/infodemic#tab=tab_1

Žižek, S. (2020). There Will Be No Return to Normality after COVID. We Are Entering a Post-Human Era & Will Have to Invent a New Way of Life. *RT*, 8 December. https://www.rt.com/op-ed/508940-normality-covid-pandemic-return/

3 'Pandemic strategy' is an oxymoron in a neoliberal world

Rodrick Wallace and Deborah Wallace

1   Introduction

Many of us who grew up during the worst of the Cold War remember participating in grade-school nuclear attack 'survival drills'. These involved being instructed to cower under our desks in 'duck and cover' mode until an 'all clear' signal was announced, allowing us to emerge unscathed into the Brave New Post Attack World. Into the early 1960s, ludicrous 'civil defense drills' were held in New York City, the prime US nuclear war target, until organized civil disobedience brought them to a halt.

Such drills might well have saved a comparatively large number of individuals from immediate demise, although the initial loss of life in a nuclear exchange would still be immense. By 1962, Ervin et al. (1962) had realistically analyzed the outcome of such a nuclear exchange, in particular, a 10-weapon, 56 megaton strike on the US city of Boston. The initial attack was supposed to kill some 2.2 million – not an insignificant loss – triggering, however, a larger series of events:

> The longer-term survival of human populations after this ecologic upheaval would be precarious. Even assuming an intact social structure and the maintenance of a functioning workforce, agriculture, particularly domestic animals, would be all but destroyed. Before malnutrition became a major medical concern, however, the threat of epidemic infectious disease would be raised by the fact that bacteria, fungi, viruses and insects would survive the effects of radiation. The ultimate size of these populations in the absence of challenge by their natural enemies is difficult to estimate.

At present writing, the saner parts of the world obey constraints of face masks, social distancing, and periodic isolating lockdowns, confronted by the emergent infection COVID-19 that has already killed more than the NEJM's (New England Journal of Medicine) predicted 2.2 million fatalities from a nuclear attack (Glazer et al., 1962). With hope and trepidation, we await the medical miracle of the RNA vaccines. Indeed, the global one percenters are now getting their shots, and availability will eventually percolate down the social hierarchy (see Dare & Kingsbury's chapter for a discussion of ethical issues pertaining to vaccination). It has taken the better part of a year to manufacture and test those vaccines, let alone distribute them as needed.

There is, however, a parallel event that has only occasionally made it into the collective consciousness: the African Swine Fever (ASF) pandemic (OIE, 2020). This emergent infection, concentrated in hog factory farms, does not have COVID-19's 2 percent fatality rate. ASF, which is highly contagious, kills half of the animals infected. Hog immune systems are so close to human that there are realistic plans to 'farm' organs in hogs for human transplant (for example Weintraub, 2019).

What would happen if ASF jumped species, highly contagious, with a fatality rate of 20–50 percent? We know such things are possible and have examples of other viral infections.

Wallace and Wallace (2015) describe something of the underlying economic and power dynamics that enable such jumps:

> With the globalization of the livestock industry, the distances over which food animal populations are transported have expanded to continental and even inter-continental scales. [Food and Agriculture Organization data] shows a surge in worldwide hog exports post-1990. The upswing in livestock miles goes hand in hand with the global spread of a corporate model of vertically integrated husbandry associated with farm consolidation and increases in head count per farm . . . By way of structural adjustment programmes and free-trade agreements, large-scale agribusinesses are moving company operations to the global South and Eastern Europe to take advantage of cheap labour, cheap land, weak regulation, and domestic production hobbled in favour of heavily subsidized agro-exporting. As a result, livestock and poultry monocultures of limited diversity and inherently dubious immunity are being raised right up against what have been long documented as reservoirs of multiple endemic pathogens, including year-round circulating strains of influenza.

There are other mechanisms. These include the corporate land grabs that gave birth to 'neoliberal Ebola' in West Africa (Wallace & Wallace, 2016), and the capital-led deforestation that has spread vector-borne diseases across much of the 'developing' world (for example Wallace et al., 2018). Others involve industrialized expansion of traditional medicines, the widening use of pesticides in previously pristine environments – forcing bat populations into new, extended, ecoregimes – and so on. All such mechanisms are, of course, likely to be greatly exacerbated by the burdens of climate change following rising carbon dioxide levels, a process fiercely defended by the fossil fuel industry.

It is worth exploring the underlying ecology of longstanding relations between pathogens and animal populations in the context of agroecological upheavals.

Biologists have an axiom that a good parasite does not kill its host but lives off its host while allowing its host to reproduce. A win/win situation. We think of parasites as multicellular creatures such as tapeworms or liver flukes, but many microbes live in hosts, gaining a safe haven and nutrition without giving much in return at the individual level. SIV, the monkey version of HIV, is such a microbe. The coronaviruses that have caused public health threats (Middle East Respiratory Syndrome, Severe Acute Respiratory Syndrome and COVID-19) originated in bats and do not cause the individual bats serious problems as long as the bats are healthy. The virus that causes Ebola also lives in bats in a similar arrangement.

These good parasites may help host populations by killing off only those too weakened to maintain immunity to the microbe. Bats that live in caves are resource limited with respect to housing and insect prey. The bats hosting the original coronavirus that causes COVID-19 (Chinese horseshoe bats) likely have a harem reproductive structure with a few males actually fathering babies, each male having several mates. Thus, some males may fall into the category of 'excess'. The hibernation-and-reproduction cycle of these bats exposes the males to a window of heightened vulnerability to their virus loads: during peak reproductive time, the immune system is at its lowest. Thus, the viruses may crop the males that cannot mount an immune defense during this time and leave the reproductive field to indeed the fittest (Kawamoto, 2003).

Over many reproductive cycles, the bat and the virus co-evolved to benefit each other at the population level.

Wild waterfowl such as ducks and gulls may carry low-pathogenic avian influenza (LPAI) without symptoms. These carriers can infect domestic fowl. LPAI can mutate into high-pathogenic avian influenza and cause disease and death to domestic flocks. Like the coronaviruses in bats, LPAI causes little or no problem to the wild host. Swine influenza (H1N1) has not been studied enough in wild swine populations to allow any conclusions about whether it causes disease or few or no symptoms.

African swine fever is not swine flu. It is caused by a DNA virus and has soft ticks as its vector in its area of origin. It had a long-stable relationship with African warthogs and soft ticks. With the introduction of domestic pigs to Africa, the virus shifted to that population and no longer required ticks as a vector reservoir. In fact, in all new areas such as Europe and Asia, transmission is direct without a vector. It causes very high rates of death among domestic hogs but has not caused any known cases in humans (Beltran-Alcrudo et al., 2017).

Thus, we can see a pattern: long-established relationships between a virus and its wild host often result in no symptoms in the host as long as the host is healthy. Transmission from the wild host to other animals and humans, caused by new patterns of contact between the original host populations and these other populations, results in disease and often high fatality rates to the new hosts.

Here, we will further focus on factory farming and related 'economies of scale' that neoliberal corporate agroecologies impose through their inherently confiscatory market strategies. See Wallace (2016, 2020) for details of the corporate global restructuring of agriculture that strips out sterilizing variations in time, space and genetic structure, and offloads the resulting risks to small holders. We will have more to say on those dynamics below, but must first explore something of the difference between pandemics a hundred years ago and those now emerging.

The arguments that follow use increasingly detailed mathematical models to explore social, ecological and infection dynamics. The first such, based on the classic Kendall model, condenses space and social structure, taking the 1918–19 pandemic as a benchmark. The next section elaborates the social and spatial dynamics of contagion in the context of stochastic variation, and a third explores individually the particular effects of temporal, spatial and genetic variability on infection spread. The spirit of these exercises is that of the theoretical ecologist Pielou (1977), who insisted that the central purpose of mathematical models of complex ecological phenomena is not to find answers, but to raise questions for empirical and observational exploration. That is very much the purpose here. The questions we raise, however, are well beyond fundamental.

2   The magnitude of the challenge

Taubenberger and Morens (2006) estimate that the 1918–19 influenza pandemic infected about a third of the world's population of 1.5 billion, providing a benchmark against which to estimate penetrance of a similar pathogen under similar travel patterns, but at current levels of population, say 7 billion. The tool for this is the standard mathematical model of an infection with removal (Bailey, 1975). Assume N individuals in the population. At time t, $X(t)$ of them are susceptible to infection, $Y(t)$ infective and $Z(t)$ 'removed' by immunization or incapacitation. The standard dynamic expressions are

$$N = X(t)+Y(t)+Z(t)$$
$$dX/dt = -\beta XY$$
$$dY/dt = (\beta X-\gamma)Y \tag{3.1}$$
$$dZ/dt = \gamma Y$$

Here, β is the rate of infection, γ the removal rate and $\rho \equiv \gamma/\beta$ determines the condition for epidemic collapse. If, at time $t = 0$, $X(0) < \rho$, no infection can propagate. Bailey (1975, Eq. 6.22) demonstrates how, if I is the proportion of all susceptible individuals eventually infected – assuming a very small number initially infected and a large N – and defining a 'critical population ratio' $S \equiv N/\rho$ – then

$$N/\rho = S = -\log(1-I)/I \tag{3.2}$$

having the solution

$$I = S + \frac{L_W(-S\exp[-S])}{S} \tag{3.3}$$

where L_W is the Lambert W-function of order zero. This function solves the relation $x = L_W(x) \exp[L_W(x)]$, and is tabulated in a number of computer algebra programs. However, this relation is also the size of the giant component of a percolation on a random network (Gandolfi, 2013). Figure 3.1 shows I as a function of S.

Taking the 1918–19 example as a foundation, with some 1/3 of 1.5 billion becoming infected, the critical population is about 1.23 billion. At a population of 7 billion, the infection penetrance rises from 0.33 to an ultimate value – after a long time – greater than 0.99, *assuming 1918–19 contact probabilities.*

Untrammeled air transport is, of course, a far more efficient agent for disease spread than sea, rail or road transport, as efficient as these have proven to be.

We are, then, only at the very first stages of a long siege from COVID-19, temporarily held in abeyance by lockdowns and other 'non-pharmaceutical interventions', while we await a medical miracle vaccine.

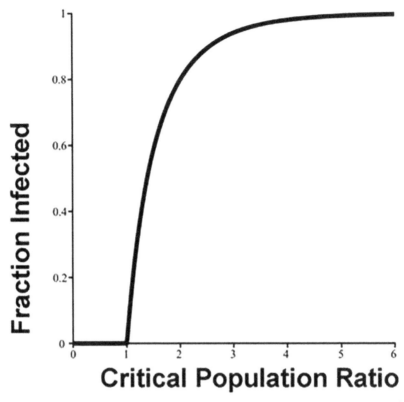

Note: For the 1918–19 influenza pandemic, about one third of the total population of 1.5 billion became infected. This implies a critical population of 1.23 billion. The 2015 population is about seven billion, suggesting a ration N/ρ of about 5.7, leading to a pandemic penetrance of greater than 0.99, assuming 1918–19 contact probabilities.

Figure 3.1   The total fraction of an initially susceptible population infected as a function of the critical population ratio $S = /\rho$

3   Pandemic spread

Once an emerging infection enters a nation's travel network, how does it actually spread?

For well over a hundred fifty years, geographers have studied how fads, rumors, technical innovations and epidemics spread across the globe, within countries, communities and smaller social groupings. There are, in general,

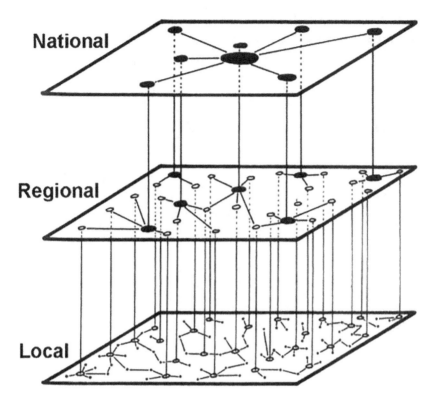

National

Regional

Local

Source: Adapted from Abler et al. (1971).

Figure 3.2   National, regional and local levels of diffusion

three levels for such spread within a nation, as illustrated in Figure 3.2, adapted from the textbook by Abler et al. (1971).

The slowest and most deceptive stage in pandemic spread – the top layer of the figure – is 'hierarchical diffusion'. In this process, a few infections enter a nation's largest cities by ordinary mechanisms – now usually air travel – where disease spreads rapidly, particularly within disadvantaged and marginalized populations forced to live under crowded and often unhealthy conditions. This community spread is usually unnoticed until it is too late because of neglect. The infection then explodes within the largest cities, and is subsequently transmitted from the larger to the smaller via air, rail, highway and boat transit. This process takes some time, and smaller cities and geographically removed rural areas may have the illusion that they will not be affected by the explosions of infection in the bigger cities.

The second level of pandemic spread, significantly more rapid than the first, is from a central city into its surrounding suburbs, along the daily back and forth of the journey to work and other city/suburb trips such as shopping, entertainment, worship and family visits. This process takes place along road and rail routes, and is illustrated by the second layer of the figure. The pattern has often been described as 'a spreading wine stain on a tablecloth', and will ultimately enmesh even the most affluent suburban enclaves.

The third level of spread – the bottom of the figure – is closely personal and much, much faster than the other two levels. It involves infection along the social networks that connect people face to face within families, friendships, schools, workplaces, shops, transport venues and so on. The technical term is 'network diffusion'. It is here that such policies as mask wearing and social distancing interrupt chains of infection, although these policies also work to deter spread at the two higher levels.

Somewhat counterintuitively, following Gould and Wallace (1994), the spread of infection on a network of interacting geographic, social group, composite or other, sites, both between and within them, can be characterized at a nonequilibrium steady state by an equilibrium distribution μ_i 'per unit area' A_i of a Markov process, where the 'areas' (which may or may not be simple geographic domains) A_i scale with the different 'size' of each network node. These nodes are assumed to be distinguishable by the scale variable A_i as well as by its 'position' i or by an associated probability-of-contact matrix (PCM). The PCM is then normalized to a stochastic matrix $\mathbf{Q}$ having unit row sums. This permits calculation, in a standard manner, of the equilibrium distribution vector as $\mu = \mu\mathbf{Q}$.

There is, we assume, a vector set of dimensionless network flows $\chi_t^i, i = 1, \dots, n$ at time t, determined as

$$\chi_t^i = g(t, \mu_i / A_i) \tag{3.4}$$

where i is the index of a particular node, χ_t^i is the corresponding dimensionless scaled ith infection rate 'signal', t the time and g an appropriate function. Recall that μ_i is defined as the left eigenvector $\mu = \mu\mathbf{Q}$ of the stochastic matrix $\mathbf{Q}$. This has been calculated as the network PCM between regions, normalized to unit row sums.

The matrix $\mathbf{Q}$ breaks out the underlying network topology, a fixed between-and-within travel or other contact configuration weighted by usage that is assumed to change relatively slowly on the timescale of observation compared with the time needed to approach the nonequilibrium steady state distribution.

The χ has been expressed in dimensionless form, g, t so that A must itself be rewritten as dimensionless as well. Thus, for the monotonic increasing function G

$$\chi_\tau^i = G[\tau, \frac{\mu_i}{A_i} \times A_\tau] \tag{3.5}$$

A_τ is the value of a *characteristic area* representing the spread of the infection at a (dimensionless) characteristic time $\tau = t/T_0$.

The expression for G may be quite complicated, including other dimensionless variates for each individual geographic node i. The central point is that the characteristic 'area' A_τ grows according to a stochastic process, even though G may be a deterministic mixmaster driven by systematic local probability of contact or other flow patterns.

An example.

The characteristic area of an infection outbreak cannot grow indefinitely, so there must be a 'carrying capacity' for the geographic, social, composite or other, network under study. Call it $K > 0$. The appropriate stochastic differential equation describing system dynamics is then

$$dA_\tau = [\mu\rho A_\tau (1 - A_\tau / K)]d\tau + \sigma A_\tau dW_\tau \tag{3.6}$$

Here, ρ represents a policy-driven 'smoothing' index across an initially highly irregular mosaic enterprise, subdivided by dynamic land-use modes, punctuated time frames, population genetic variabilities and so on. We will provide some more explicit models below.

Application of the Itô chain rule for stochastic differential equations (Protter, 2005) to $\log(A)$, as a consequence of the added Itô correction factor and the Jensen inequality for a concave function, gives

$$E(A) \to 0, \; \mu\rho < \sigma^2/2$$
$$E(A) \geq K(1 - \frac{\sigma^2}{2\mu\rho}), \; \mu\rho \geq \sigma^2/2 \tag{3.7}$$

While zero can be reached as a stochastic limit of the characteristic area below the critical smoothing value, above that, the infection becomes endemic, and, as smoothing increases, may attain its greatest possible value as a full-scale pandemic.

The graph of Equation 3.7 is quite similar to Figure 3.1, for obvious reasons.

In sum, to put the cart a little before the horse, neoliberal or colonial smoothing of 'outback' land use practices will cause sporadic disease outbreaks that would die out rapidly and be limited both socially and geographically to become either endemic or of significant spatial extent. These are then entrained into larger travel patterns and deposited in central places, where they incubate and then spread explosively down and across social and economic hierarchies.

We now focus more specifically on the neoliberal agribusiness model, involving 'economies of scale' that strip out stochastic variabilities of time, place and genetic structure characteristic of more traditional agricultural practices.

4   Factory farming as pandemic incubator

The political economy of neoliberal corporate agribusiness – 'Big Ag' – is well known and has been described in detail elsewhere (for example Wallace, 2016, 2020; Wallace and Wallace, 2016; Wallace et al., 2018; and references therein). The essential features involve the imposition of economies of scale at all scales and levels of organization, permitting undercutting of more traditional or established local agricultural ecosystems. The subsequent de-facto economic monopoly then permits imposition of 'all the traffic will bear' pricing, in concert with restructuring that reduces local smallholders from independent operators to powerless, dependent clients forced to bear the most risky aspects of corporate condensation.

Our particular focus will be on the burdens Big Ag 'factory farming' of hogs and chickens places on global public health. Other aspects of Big Ag are, of course, also of central interest. These include, but are not limited to, the conversion of traditional highly mixed agricultural ecologies into monocrop, monogenetic plantations, associated neocolonial land grabs, deforestation, exploitation of wild populations, acceleration of global warming and so on.

Here, we will unpack the implications of Equation 3.7, studying the particular dynamics of stochastic sterilization in time, place and genetic structure.

Temporal variability

For the earliest stage of an infection in a population of susceptible individuals – the 'explosion' before intervention or 'removal' at time t,

$$dN/dt \approx \alpha N(t) \qquad\qquad (3.8)$$

Here, N is the infected population and α is the rate of growth of the infection, where $N(t)$ increases exponentially as

$$N(t) = N_0 \exp[\alpha t] \qquad\qquad (3.9)$$

The stochastic version of this is a stochastic differential differential equation

$$dN_t = \alpha N_t dt + \sigma N_t dW_t \qquad\qquad (3.10)$$

The second term imposes a volatility under a Brownian white noise dW_t, a random signal with equal power within a fixed bandwidth at any center of frequency. The magnitude of noise effect is through σ.

Applying the Itô chain rule (Protter, 2005), a stochastic version of computing the derivative of the composition of two or more functions, to $\log[N]$ gives

$$d\log[N_t] = (\alpha - \frac{\sigma^2}{2})dt + \sigma dW_t \qquad\qquad (3.11)$$

The term $-\sigma^2/2$ is the 'correction factor'. Heuristically, from this we can write

$$E(N_t) \rightarrow N_0 \exp[(\alpha - \sigma^2/2)t] \qquad\qquad (3.12)$$

If $\sigma^2/2 > \alpha$, an outbreak will eventually be driven to extinction.

For 'colored' noise, having nonuniform spectral densities, similar results emerge from invoking the Doleans-Dade exponential (Protter, 2006).

Wallace et al. (2018) expand this analysis to multidimensional vector-borne diseases, where there are both host and vector populations. For the most part, sufficient variability will drive the infection to extinction.

In sum, a sufficiently large stochastic variation 'sterilizes' disease outbreaks, our first parallel to Equation 3.7.

Spatial variability

Here, we follow the classic exposition of Murray (1989, Sec. 14.8). In a single space dimension x, we take $N(x, t)$ as the number of infected individuals at location x for t, and write a 'diffusion equation' for the very first part of an epidemic:

$$\partial N(x,t)/\partial t = \mu \partial^2 N(x,t)/\partial x^2 + \alpha N(x,t) \tag{3.13}$$

It is possible to expand the solution to this equation as a spatial Fourier series. This leads to a time dependence proportional to

$$\exp[(\alpha - C^2 \mu / L^2)t] \tag{3.14}$$

Here, α is the growth rate, μ the coefficient of spatial diffusion and C is a constant near 1 that depends on the dimension of the diffusion. The essential point is that infection dies out if the patch size L is less than the critical length $L_c = C\sqrt{\mu/\alpha}$. This leads to a second 'spatial temperature' analog $T_L \equiv 1/L_c = \sqrt{\alpha/\mu}/C$.

Equation 3.7 represents a generalized version of this result that can be applied to diffusion of infection on a 'commuting field' linking network nodes.

Genetic variability

The effect of host genetic structure on epidemic emergence and propagation has been a topic of study for some time (for example O'Brien and Everman, 1988; King and Lively, 2010).

Lively (2010) presents a stochastic model under a fixed reproductive cycle, for example, annual birthing or, in the factory farm context, market-driven turnover.

The model assumes the number of infected hosts having the ith genotype at time $t + 1$ is

$$I_{i(t+1)} = g_{i(t+1)} N_{t+1} P_{i(t+1)} \tag{3.15}$$

Here, $g_{i(t+1)}$ is the frequency of the ith host genotype at time $t + 1$, N_{t+1} is the total number of hosts at time $t + 1$ and $P_{i(t+1)}$ is the probability of infection for the ith host genotype at time $t + 1$.

Under a Poisson distribution, P is 1 minus the zero class $\exp[-\lambda]$, with λ the mean number of matching spores that contact each host.

The probability of ith host genotype infection at $t + 1$ becomes

$$P_{i(t+1)} = 1 - \exp[-\lambda] = 1 - \exp\left[-BI_{i(t)}/N_{t+1}\right] \tag{3.16}$$

Here, $I_{i(t)}$ is the number of infected hosts with the ith genotype at time t and B is the number of infectious propagules produced by each infection that make contact with different hosts, imposing an upper limit on secondary infections.

Under the model, a single infected individual, having genotype i, is introduced into the population of hosts at time t. Then, $I_{i(t)} = 1$, and the number of secondary infections – the infamous R_0 – becomes

$$R_{0i} = g_{i(t+1)}N_{t+1}\left(1 - \exp\left[-B/N_{t+1}\right]\right) \tag{3.17}$$

The propagation condition is then

$$g_{i(t+1)}N_{t+1} > \frac{1}{\left(1 - \exp\left[-B/N_{t+1}\right]\right)} \tag{3.18}$$

For $N \to \infty$, Equation (3.17) implies

$$R_{0i} = g_i B > 1$$
$$B > \frac{1}{g_i} \tag{3.19}$$

Consequently, given a large population, if the single-strain infection reduces the fitness and the frequency of the susceptible host genotype over time, the infection will die out when g_i becomes less than $1/B$.

Lively's (2010) model further implies that, if the pathogen is introduced by migration at a high rate, there can be multiple coexisting strains of the infective agent. This produces a mean value for R_0 as

$$<R_0> = \frac{\sum R_{0i}}{G} = \frac{N_{t+1}\left(1 - \exp\left[-B/N_{t+1}\right]\right)}{G} \to \frac{B}{G} \tag{3.20}$$

for N large, where G is the number of genotypes in the host population.

Lively (2010) concludes

> Thus, all else being equal, the spread and persistence of infection should more easily occur in genetically homogeneous populations.

The implications for variability in time, space and genetics are clear. Increased 'stochasticity temperatures' leading to disease control can be regionally planned. Mechanisms that include crop rotation, agrobiodiversity and ecological pest control can be imposed by market regulation and trade/tax structures and policies (for example Chappell, 2018).

In sum, sufficiently mosaic agroecologies at large spatial and population scales, by virtue of their rich environmental stochastic variabilities, will preempt – in effect 'burn out' – most large-scale diseases before they emerge. Such agroecologies are feasible with appropriate government regulation and support.

5   Discussion

The Anglo-American scholar of military strategy Colin S. Gray, toward the end of his masterclass *Theory of Strategy* (Gray, 2018), writes

> Strategy's general theory does not apply to the nuclear dimension of security because there can be no meaningful nuclear strategy. If used in warfare, nuclear weapons would be most likely too powerful to serve political purposes. Of course, plans for nuclear use can be, and are, devised and certainly could be implemented, but what next? . . . [S]trategy is all about the consequences of action (or inaction). Anyone purporting to write about the contextual terra incognita of nuclear strategy should pause to reflect [that] . . . the cardinal virtue of strategy must be prudence.

Gray was the principal architect of US nuclear policy during the Reagan Administration, and his experience of a strategic 'engineering curve' on these matters is notable.

As Ervin et al. (1962) (and many others) so clearly foresaw early on, there can be no rational 'nuclear strategy'.

Can there be a rational 'pandemic strategy' designed to isolate and insulate current neoliberal agribusiness enterprise? Can we institute a rapid-response biomedical fire brigade that stamps out emerging infection whenever and wherever it appears? A fire brigade that, failing to prevent epidemic spread, fast tracks advanced molecular biological approaches to development of a vaccine in time to prevent mass death? A pandemic fire suppression program that always works?

The emergence of HIV from the colonially brutalized African continent provides a singular counterexample. The virus' rapid rate of mutation precludes vaccine development, and engineering effective antiretrovirals proved exceedingly difficult.

The emergence of ASF provides another counterexample. As of 2022, there is no effective vaccine, and the fatality rate among hog populations is about one-half.

Wallace et al. (2020), in the context of COVID-19, describe the dilemma of firefighting itself in these terms,

> . . . [If] firefighters are given sufficient resources, under normal conditions, most fires, most often, can be contained with minimal casualties and property destruction. However, that containment is critically dependent on a far less romantic, but no less heroic enterprise [than active firefighting], the persistent, ongoing, regulatory efforts that limit building hazard through code development and enforcement, and that also ensure firefighting, sanitation, and building preservation resources are supplied to all at needed levels.
>
> If industry lobbyists are permitted to weaken building codes, for example allowing the use of aluminum wiring and polyvinyl chloride (PVC) electrical insulation and construction materials in places of business or residences (Wallace, 1990), if 'demographic engineers' are allowed to cut firefighting resources in communities of color with the intent of dispersing voting blocs (Wallace & Wallace, 1998), then there are deadly consequences. Under such conditions, individual fires very often cannot be contained, and indeed, can create 'South Bronx' fire/abandonment epidemics that consume vast stretches of urban landscape, triggering massive loss of life, both directly, and by long-term 'avalanche' social and public health mechanisms (again, Wallace & Wallace, 1998).
>
> In sum, code development-and-enforcement that prevents fires is far preferable to actual firefighting, necessary as that may always be.

Firefighting models for pandemic prevention and address are grossly inadequate without constraining the neoliberal agribusiness and land use structures and practices primarily responsible for pandemic disease. Such a program would necessarily involve significant alterations in the power relations between groups within civil society. It is, after all, the breakdown of what US economist J.K. Galbraith called 'countervailing forces' that has led us down a neoliberal road toward a neo-serfdom. Such 'countervailing forces' keep quasimonoplies from reducing society at large to feudalism. They include labor unions, human rights organizations, environmental groups, public health associations and so on.

The neoliberal World Order, however, now stands on the brink of a Justinian abyss, much as did the institution of European serfdom in 1300, on the eve of the Black Plague.

Governmental responses to the COVID-19 pandemic varied widely from the delayed response at the point of origin (Wuhan), which abetted the hierarchical diffusion worldwide, to the rapid and strong policies in New Zealand and South Korea, which quashed the first wave. Governmental response grows out of socioeconomic, political and cultural roots and reflects human strengths and weaknesses. The 1960s ads for the Negro College Fund in the United States adopted the slogan: 'We are only as strong as our weakest link' and showed a chain with a broken link. Because of the extreme contagion of several spillover diseases and because some feature both asymptomatic infection and infectious asymptomatic incubation periods before symptoms develop, delayed and weak responses by even a few governments threaten the entire world with the pandemic. COVID-19 featured widespread community spread before detection in country after country from China to the United States.

We have all witnessed the trade-off between public health and socioeconomic values in governmental struggles to contain the pandemic within the jurisdictional borders. Fear of the unknown and of the severity of the threat may paralyze decision makers who then extend the delay and weaken the response with these trade-offs. Governmental officials are, after all, staring death in the face, their own deaths and unknown numbers of deaths of their constituents. They are also in fear of their own political death. We have witnessed how this delayed and weak response failed to stem the contagion. Delay and temporizing of the response may be inevitable in governments of fragmented societies afflicted with internal strife over basic values. This decisional delay piles on top of the detection delay that allows the disease to spread widely.

Containment, whether by non-pharmaceutical means or by new vaccines, costs society economically and socially. We have witnessed the unequal burden of illness, death, exposure, job loss, housing loss, famine and lack of health care: inevitable outcomes of a colonialist neo-liberal structure. Thus, the originators of the pandemics externalize the true costs of their industries onto society, which concentrates these costs in the marginalized population sectors. Furthermore, the pharmaceutical means of containment and of healing the sick channels societal resources into industry hands and accelerates the accumulation of wealth into the top tier and away from the bottom.

Furthermore, the originators of the pandemics often externalize the ecological and environmental health costs of their industries. In Nigeria, communities around the oil fields operated by Western companies suffered from pollution of their water. Those who tried to organize against this health hazard were imprisoned and sometimes killed, but Western societies failed to react strongly to this outrage.

The originators of the pandemics often conduct land grabs or coerced consolidation of independent small farms into large cooperatives. The small farmers end up receiving very low compensation for their products, whether palm oil or chickens, and bearing the brunt of the local risks such as spillover infections. Although Western societies were informed of these infringements of land rights, they failed to react strongly to these outrages.

Perhaps the pandemics visited on Western societies follow the ancient myths about plagues as indicators of corrupt leaders of corrupt societies. Perhaps the pandemics are just paybacks for fattening on the suffering of the powerless in economically colonized countries. Perhaps the pandemics may finally offer at least a glimmer of understanding that the societies that originate these sins against nature and humanity must atone for them and stop them (see also Lambert in this volume).

We end with exploration of some of the cultural and political 'research blindspots' hindering pandemic prevention across the globe.

The dominant research paradigm in response to COVID-19 – and to the threat of future pandemics – revolves around control measures once the disease has entered a new area. Epidemiological mathematical modeling, in particular, has flourished and dictated policies for non-pharmaceutical prevention. Current discussion focuses on 'more and better' such models, adapting techniques used in climate change studies that focus on outcome distributions given random parameter variations (Adam, 2020).

Vaccine development and distribution has also gained vast resources, as did study of the physiology of the disease and its short- and long-term injuries. This last has led to improvements in health care (see McDonagh's chapter on international vaccine diplomacy). Upstream research questions, however, remain largely unaddressed.

However, prevention by avoidance of 'spillover' has been starved of resources. Ecological data acquisition on the host animals that often show few or no symptoms from infections, economic geographic data acquisition on human actions that result in spillover and politico-economic data acquisition on the forces behind these human actions receive little or no funding. These topics actually may be unofficially banned by governments seeking to develop industrial agriculture, extractive industries and industrialization of traditional medicine.

Apart from such academic research, developmental land grabs continue to dissolve enforcement of environmental protection and of human rights in the face of economic colonialism and governmental corruption. Research into education of passive and hostile white and Asian populations may require dangerous experimentation of engagement with potentially violent sectors. It may require risking prison or death. Without broader understanding and acceptance of how spillover events occur, and of the likely future waves of pandemics with high fatality rates, none of the research that has been done and that will be done can save humankind from massive fatality rates and rates of long-term serious sequelae from disease.

References

Abler, R., J. Adams, P. Gould, 1971, *Spatial Organization: The Geographer's View of the World*, Prentice-Hall, New Jersey.

Adam, D., 2020, What COVID pandemic forecasters can learn from climate models, *Nature* 587:533–4.

Bailey, N.T.J., 1975, *The Mathematical Theory of Infectious Diseases and its Applications*. Hafner, New York.

Beltran-Alcrudo, D., M. Arias, C. Gallardo, S. Kramer, M. Penrith, 2017, African swine fever: Detection and diagnosis – A manual for veterinarians. *FAO Animal Production and Health Manual No. 19*, Rome: Food and Agriculture Organization, United Nations.

Chappell, M.J., 2018, *Beginning to End Hunger: Food and the Environment in Belo Horizonte, Brazil, and Beyond*, University of California Press, Berkeley.

Ervin, F., J. Glazer, S. Aronow, D. Nathan, R. Coleman, N. Avery, et al., 1962, Human and ecologic effects in Massachusetts of an assumed thermonuclear attack on the United States, *New England Journal of Medicine* 266:1127–37.

Gandolfi, A., 2013, Percolation methods for SEIR epidemics on graphs. In V. Rao, R. Durvasula (Eds.), *Dynamic Models of Infectious Diseases: Volume 2*, Non vector-borne diseases (Chap. 2, pp. 31–58), Springer, New York.

Gould, P., R. Wallace, 1994, Spatial structures and scientific paradoxes in the AIDS pandemic, *Geografiska Annaler B* 76:105–16.

Gray, C.S., 2018, *Theory of Strategy, Oxford University Press*, New York.

Kawamoto, K., 2003, Endocrine control of reproductive activity in hibernation bats, *Zoological Science* 20:1057–69.

King, K., C. Lively, 2012, Does genetic diversity limit disease spread in natural host populations? *Heredity* 109:199–203.

Lively C., 2010, The effect of host genetic diversity on disease spread, *The American Naturalist* 175:E149–E152 (E-Note)

Murray, J., 1989, *Mathematical Biology*, Springer, New York.

O'Brien, S., J. Evermann, 1988, Interactive inuence of infectious disease and genetic diversity in natural populations, *Trends in Ecology and Evolution* 3:254–9.

OIE 2020 https://www.oie.int/en/animal-health-in-the-world/animal-diseases/african-swine-fever/

Pielou, E.C., 1977, *Mathamatical Ecology*, Wiley, New York.

Protter, P., 2005, *Stochastic Integration and Differential Equations*, 2nd ed, Springer, New York.

Taubenberger J.K., D.M. Morens, 2006, 1918 Influenza: The mother of all pandemics. *Emerg Infect Dis.* 1:15–22. https://doi: 10.3201/eid1201.050979. PMID: 16494711

Wallace, D., 1990, *In the Mouth of the Dragon: Toxic Fires in the Age of Plastics*, Avery, New York.

Wallace, D., R. Wallace, 1998, *A Plague on Your Houses*, Verso, New York.

Wallace, R., L.F. Chaves, L. Bergmann, C. Ayres, L. Hogerwerf, R. Kock, R.G. Wallace, 2018, *Clear-Cutting Disease Control: Capital-Led Deforestation, Public Health Austerity, and Vector-Borne Infection*, Springer, New York.

Wallace, R., R.G. Wallace, 2015, Blowback: New formal perspectives on agriculturally driven pathogen evolution and spread, *Epidemiology and Infection* 143:2068–80.

Wallace, R.G., 2016, *Big Farms Make Big Flu: Dispatches on Infectious Disease, Agribusiness, and the Nature of Science*, Monthly Review Press, New York.

Wallace, R.G., A. Liebman, L.F. Chaves, R. Wallace, 2020, *Dead Epidemiologists: On the Origins of COVID-19*, Monthly Review Press, New York.

Wallace, R.G., R. Wallace (Eds.) 2016, *Neoliberal Ebola: Modeling Disease Emergence From Finance to Forest to Farm*, Springer, New York.

Weintraub, K., 2019, https://www.technologyreview.com/2019/11/01/132110/meet-the-pigs-that-could-solve-the-human-organ-transplant-crises/

4   COVID-19 and Swedish exceptionalism

Richey Wyver

Introduction

The Swedish response to the COVID-19 crisis has been reported internationally with a mix of morbid fascination and awe, usually through a lens of Sweden being a progressive, liberal home of human rights, equality and democracy. Over time, the devastating impacts of Swedish policy and staggering death rates may have led to an increase in criticism, but, in general, reporting has tended to swing between two extremes of 'has Sweden got it all wrong?' and 'was Sweden right all along?' (Daly, 2020; Jackson, 2020).

Both extremes share the premise of there being a uniquely Swedish way of approaching the crisis, and that this approach is radical and exceptional. It is also portrayed as being calculated, organized and universally embraced by the people. Yet intrigue arises from the conundrum of the Swedish approach – and Sweden – being celebrated for liberty, democracy and equality, yet seemingly accepting a high level of deaths, particularly among the elderly and immigrant communities. Sweden has been persistently near the top of tables of per capita death rates, and has on occasion peaked as having the highest reported death rates globally (Cuthbertson, 2020). By the end of October 2021, Sweden had officially recorded 14 982 (Anderson, 2020) deaths, at a rate of 1471 deaths per 1 million people (worldometers.com, 2021). This death rate is significantly higher than that of neighbouring states with comparable Nordic welfare state political traditions: Denmark and Norway had recorded 456 and 163 deaths per million people, respectively, in the same time frame (worldometers.com, 2021). Despite this, within Sweden open criticism of the approach to handling the crisis has seemingly been minimal.

In this chapter, I discuss how a fixation with the idea of a uniquely 'Swedish way' and a myth of Swedish exceptionalism is reflected in international reporting and in Swedish policy, and the significance of this. This chapter is centred around the question of what we can learn about Swedish exceptionalism from the COVID-19 response and the international perceptions of it.

A Swedish way?

The Swedish COVID-19 strategy has been one of herd immunity, the fundamental premise of which is allowing the virus to spread through non-vulnerable sections of the population in the hope of building up a collective level of immunity (Habib, 2020). This strategy has meant that Sweden has avoided a formal lockdown, and most business have been able to remain open, including bars and gyms. An emphasis has been placed on the expectation of individuals to act responsibly and follow recommended behavioural guidelines, as members of an intelligent and informed population that can be trusted to make the 'right' decisions (Anderson, 2020).

Officially, the Swedish government has denied that they are pursuing a strategy of herd immunity, yet as Kelly Bjorklund points out in *Foreign Policy* (2020), this has become an accepted truth in international perceptions. Additionally, the Swedish strategy *does* exemplify one of herd immunity, and recently declassified emails between state epidemiologist Anders Tegnell, the popular public face of Sweden's COVID-19 response, and other officials clearly reveal that herd immunity was categorically stated as an objective and an approach, with an acknowledgement that it would entail a number of deaths along the way. Such a strategy was also recommended to other states, with Tegnell advising his Finnish counterpart, Mika Salminen, that people should be allowed to become infected with COVID-19, and that schools should be kept open 'to reach herd immunity more quickly' (Bjorklund, 2020).

The Swedish strategy is supposedly built around civic trust, a mutual trust between the citizens and state institutions; arguably this system of trust is the reason why most Swedes support the approach (Anderson, 2020). In addition, strong appeals to nationalism, and in the face of external criticism a narrative of Swedishness versus the world, help to bolster support and make it possible for Swedes to see critique of the COVID-19 response as an attack on Sweden and Swedishness.

Paul O'Shea, writing in *The Conversation*, explains that the Swedish strategy also draws upon a shared understanding of a concept called *folkvett*: 'In Sweden, rather than implement any mandatory restrictions, Prime Minister Stefan Lofven called on the populace to use their *folkvett* – a blend of good manners, morality, and common sense that is supposed to be innate to all good

Swedes – to follow the voluntary recommendations' (O'Shea, 2020). Behind this lies the implication that there are inherent behavioural traits in Swedish people ('innate to all good Swedes . . .') and that they can be trusted to call on these traits to behave correctly; something that other countries cannot rely on, hence their draconian laws and lockdowns.

Within Sweden, defence of the COVID-19 strategy has been staunch, and has at times taken on deep, almost aggressively nationalistic tones. The Swedish media, according to O'Shea, has played a key role in invoking and sustaining a nationalist defence of the strategy by encouraging Swedes to feel proud of living in Sweden and not under 'populist and draconian' responses to the crisis elsewhere in Europe (O'Shea, 2020). Those who have written critically about it have found themselves facing an angry backlash, however: Swedish journalist Erik Augustin Palm (2020), for example, reflects, 'I'd never received so much ad hominem vitriol from colleagues as I did after I wrote an article for *Slate* critical of the Swedish model'.

The *white* Swedish way?

The celebrated Swedish way, in terms of a uniquely Swedish way of doing and being, has proved time and again to be not one of universal equality and liberty, but one of racial segregation and exclusion. In effect, it is the *white* Swedish way (Lambert's chapter also discusses the pandemic through the optic of race). This is certainly the case when it comes to the Swedish COVID-19 response, where people of colour in Sweden, such as those of Somalian origin, have been grossly over-represented in COVID-19 death rates, and less affluent suburbs, where 'immigrant' communities tend to be concentrated, have reportedly been hardest hit by the deadly virus (Rothschild, 2020).[1]

Sweden's main broadsheet newspaper, *DN* (*Dagensnyheter*), reported in July 2020 that the first wave of COVID-19 in the European Spring had seen a 220 per cent increase in mortality rates for Swedish people over 40 who were born in Somalia, Syria and Iraq, compared with the same period in the past four years. In comparison, mortality among residents born in Sweden, the Nordic countries, the EU or North America had decreased by one per cent for 40–65 year olds, and had increased by just 19% for those older than 65 (Dagensnyheter, 2020).

Non-white communities have been indirectly and directly blamed for their higher death rates, by being accused of not understanding COVID-19 and health advice (Gustavsson, 2020). This narrative works to distance them from the Swedish national identity that is supposedly characterized by being well informed, intelligent and responsible.

The herd immunity approach inevitably results in, if not sacrificing weaker members of the national body, at least accepting their deaths. In Sweden this has been noticeable in care homes for the elderly. Some experts and commentators have attempted to direct the responsibility for these deaths away from failed state policy and onto non-white communities. For example, Johan Giesecke, the former chief epidemiologist and mentor to Tegnell, suggested in an interview that deaths in care homes were the result of staff who were 'asylum seekers' and 'refugees' not being able to understand and follow information (Gustavsson, 2020).

This idea of directing blame for the failings of herd immunity to people of colour in Sweden is reflected in international reporting too, and is clear to see in the choice of images that accompany news articles on Sweden's COVID-19 response. For example, Nathalie Rothschild's article in *Foreign Policy* (2020), which argues that immigrants are the 'hidden flaw' in Sweden's COVID-19 response, is illustrated with an image from the 2015 Syrian refugee movement into Northern Europe. It captures a chaotic scene of a crowd of people of colour ('immigrants') on a train station platform, close together, looking scruffy and confused and being directed by a policeman; a sharp contrast to the homely images of relaxed white Swedes enjoying a coffee or glass of wine outdoors in other reporting that is not focused on immigrants (see, for example, Birrell, 2020). The image, the only one to accompany the text, captures a lost and confused people, ignorant of customs and rules, rather than the careful, responsible, healthy and relaxed white Swedes in other reporting. The need for the crowd to have a directing policeman suggests a childlike ignorance. They need to be directed by the state, whereas the white Swede can be trusted to take the appropriate actions themselves, as free thinking, well-informed adults.

It addition, it is worth noting that Sweden's high death rates have also been used as an indicator of nationalistic success. State epidemiologist Anders Tegnell argued that the figures do not prove the Swedish approach is failing, but rather they are proof that 'Sweden is the best in the world in reporting the actual number of dead' (quoted in Anderson, 2020).

The Swedish approach has, unsurprisingly, done nothing to alleviate the other virus plaguing the West – racism against East Asians (and see Matthewman's chapter). Sustained and systemic racism against East Asians is, of course, nothing new, particularly in Sweden, with its troubling histories of international adoption from countries such as Korea and China (Wyver, 2020), and the on-going popularity of 'Yellow Face' performance, where white Swedish celebrities dress as 'Asians', with rice hats, false buck teeth and 'hilariously' mix Ls and Rs (Hübinette & Sjöblom, 2015; Wyver, 2015). Yet anti-Asian racism has reached a new golden age under the guise of COVID-19, with attacks on Asians being treated by some as being justified by the virus. Asians in Sweden have experienced an increase in racist taunts and violent attacks (see, for example, Bergsten, 2020; Karlsson, 2020; *The Local*, 2020). As with elsewhere, such attacks tend to relate to the perception that COVID-19 originated in China, and racial hatred is given fuel by the racialization of the virus by media and politicians.

There is a difference between reporting and reality, and while my focus here is on the perception of policy, Sweden and Swedishness, it is important to reflect on this. Looking at images in international reporting on Sweden and COVID-19, perhaps the typical scene is of young white women sipping wine outside a café. On the surface, in times of lockdown and suffering elsewhere, this signifies freedom, vitality, independence. Yet this imagery conceals the reality that older, vulnerable and sick people have had to isolate and shield themselves. It would appear, on the surface, that life has been progressing as normal in Sweden, yet this normality may just be limited to rich, young, white Swedes.

In the *New Zealand Herald* article (originally published in the UK's *Daily Mail*), 'Will Sweden Get the Last Laugh?' (Birrell, 2020), the imagery continues this theme: white, smart but casually dressed Swedish young men outside a restaurant. White people outside a bar in Stockholm; white people picnicking, drinking and hugging in a park; white people eating in an outdoor area of a restaurant, an area decorated with blue and yellow balloons (representing the colours of the Swedish flag). It is not just *normal* life, but a relaxed, fun happy life, being lived to the full, in stark contrast to depressing, lonely, strictly imposed lockdowns elsewhere. The frivolity of this life is also reflected in the headline ('laugh'). It is also a *healthy* life, out in the fresh air. These are healthy, strong fit bodies, able to enjoy life despite the virus, as their strength, health and vitality could presumably withstand COVID-19 – supposedly unlike weaker bodies elsewhere. The image outside the restaurant features an older white couple, sitting apart from the rest of their family, but still enjoying a very typically Swedish looking meal. The message is that they are Swedish (the food, the balloons, the whiteness), they are responsible and clever enough to follow health advice and exercise *folkvett* (they are sitting apart from the rest of their group), but they are hardy, resilient and healthy: the air may be chilly (they have blankets over their knees), but they are still eating out.

The fact that every single person in the images is white and we can assume Swedish, carries the myth that Swedishness equals whiteness (Lundström, 2017). Their health, happiness and strength jars against the statistics of people of colour and sick and older people dying from COVID-19. This can be read as suggesting that white Swedes could survive, even thrive, under herd immunity, whilst other could not. Indeed, Birrell's text echoes this: the white Swedes interviewed are, 'enjoying a coffee', 'dangling legs over water after a day out', and this happy, relaxed – white – people are part of a national effort, and with some of them even expressing 'adulation for Tegnell', it is an effort they are all fully on board with (Birrell, 2020).

The article mentions problems with the strategy though: COVID-19 deaths in care homes and 'migrant communities'. Care home deaths are said to make up half of all COVID-19 deaths in Sweden, and the article goes so far as to (rightly) call it a 'catastrophe': 'There was, however, catastrophe in care homes, as there was in several other nations such as Britain, Canada and Spain, which reflects years of neglect for a fragmented sector staffed by underpaid workers often flitting between different places to make ends meet' (Birrell, 2020).

The acknowledgement of the care homes catastrophe acts, in Roland Barthes's (1993) terms, as an inoculation of evil. This is where a small piece of 'evil' is acknowledged, and is used as a 'bad apple' to stand out from system. It is exposed, addressed and now fixed. Consequently, the system itself can remain unchallenged. In this case the care homes scandal is isolated from the wider problem. Note that the article ensures that this is not seen as just a Swedish issue ('as there was in several other nations'), which indicates that it is not a problem with the Swedish strategy, and that it was likely caused by staff rather than by structural issues. The staff as 'underpaid workers' in a Swedish context indicates they are 'immigrants'; in a society that is divided economically along racial lines, low paid workers with less job stability and rights are generally of an immigrant background and are often of colour (Pred, 2000).

Similarly, the placing of 'migrant communities', as being at the centre of the crisis, separates the COVID-19 problem in such communities from wider Swedish society. It enables the broader political-structural issues to go unchallenged. Headlines such as 'The Hidden Flaw in Sweden's COVID Strategy', referring to immigrants as the flaw, (Rothschild, 2020), imply that the strategy *could have* worked without the presence of immigrants.

When 'immigrant' bodies are observed externally in a desperate effort to highlight the disproportionate deaths among Swedish communities of colour, *and* when these communities and bodies are blamed for dying, there is a possibility that under the surface is an unspoken theme of race hygiene. The hidden narrative being that white Swedish 'stock' would have been able to achieve herd immunity, if it was not for the problematic presence of non-white bodies, who not only could not be trusted to behave in the appropriate Swedish way, but would physically cause the system to fail.

While there was certainly a long-held belief in there being a distinct Swedish or Nordic master race (McEachrane, 2018), speaking of a such a 'race' is no longer permissible in Swedish 'colour-blind' discourse. Yet to speak of Swedish as a nationality but exclude Swedes of colour from this by defining them as 'immigrants' regardless of immigration status, or even using the terms 'ethnic Swede' and 'native Swede' to describe a white Swedish person (Lundström, 2017), proves that Swedish is still imagined as a (white) race. It could be argued that race thinking and a shared belief in a unique race of white Swedes lingers beneath the surface of the contemporary acceptable vocabularies of nationality and ethnicity in the Swedish colour-blind discourse. What this means is that, to discuss Swedishness, a Swedish national identity, a Swedish way, is often, perhaps subconsciously, a discussion of a *White* Swedish way. In this sense a separation is made of Swedish residents into 'Immigrants' who die of COVID-19, who spread it in care homes and 'Swedes' who enjoy freedoms and who are tuned into *folkvett* and are able to follow instructions – and whose healthy, active bodies do not die from COVID-19.

Exceptionalism

Paul O'Shea, discussing Swedish and Japanese responses to the virus, reflects on the importance of national myths of exceptionalism: 'One factor that features in both the Japanese and Swedish responses is that of national exceptionalism. By exceptionalism I mean the understanding among a population that "we" are not only distinct from the rest, but in some way also superior' (O'Shea, 2020).

O'Shea argues that the nationalist and exceptionalist drive behind the Swedish strategy has left it prone to what he describes as 'Exceptionalist inertia'. While other states have managed to change tack with their strategies, adapting to new scientific advice, to changes in the virus and learning from other models, Sweden has stuck to its 'Swedish way' to the extent that face masks were still not widely used, and bars and restaurants have remained open (additionally, only recently has the idea of any sort of lockdown been initially discussed) even though, at the time of his article in December 2020, the third wave of the virus was beginning to spiral out of control (O'Shea, 2020). Connecting the success of a public health policy to a national character makes a fundamental change of course, even one based on strong evidence, difficult or even impossible (O'Shea, 2020).

An important element of Swedish exceptionalism is the image of Sweden as a uniquely 'good', anti-racist and equitable nation. This myth is shared internationally, with Sweden usually being placed at the top of various measures of 'goodness' (Siret, 2016; Anholt, 2021, The Good Country Index).

At the heart of this exceptionalism is the widely held belief that the country is a neutral actor in international affairs, and stands alone in Europe as a country without a colonial or racist past (or present, for that matter) (Gondouin, 2012; McEachrane, 2018; Pred, 2000). Olof Palme, one of the most prominent early advocates and symbols of Sweden as a globally good nation, invoked the idea of this national exceptionalism in his Christmas speech as Prime Minister in 1965: 'Democracy is firmly rooted in this country. We respect the fundamental freedoms and rights. Murky racial theories have never found a foothold here. We like to see ourselves as open-minded and tolerant' (Palme, 1968, cited in McEachrane, 2018, p. 480).[2]

Even as recently as 2008, the Swedish government maintained that Sweden was ideally suited to co-operate with Africa due to 'Sweden's lack of a colonial past in Africa' (McEachrane, 2018, p. 479). Yet in reality, Sweden was a key player in European colonial history, had its own Caribbean colony (St Bartholomy), was the pioneering home of race biology and eugenicist studies, and for many decades carried out extensive eugenics programmes (see, also, Lambert's chapter in this book).

Sweden was very much involved in the European scramble for colonies from the seventeenth century to the 1880s (McEachrane, 2018, p. 475). As with other colonial European nations, Sweden had its own African, East Indian and West Indian companies. The prosperous Swedish African Company established an important trading colony in what is now Ghana in 1650. The company traded in enslaved Africans in addition to products of slave labour such as ivory, gold and sugar (McEachrane, 2018, p. 476).

For centuries Sweden was a significant consumer of imported colonial goods produced by enslaved or indentured labour, such as plantation sugar. In his study of coloniality and race in Sweden, Michael McEachrane (2018, p. 476) argues that such consumption's role in sustaining slavery should not be overlooked: he calculates that the annual labour of 15 000 enslaved Africans was required to satisfy Swedish sugar consumption alone. Sweden was a major colonial exporter too, producing and distributing materials for use in the slave trade. Iron was Sweden's largest export, and was used for voyage irons, guns and chains and shackles, as well as for agricultural tools for colonial plantations (McEachrane, 2018, p. 476).

Sweden's colony of St Barthélemy in the Caribbean was held for almost a century. It was a free trade zone that became an epicentre of the slave trade. Gustavia, its port, was recognized as one of the most significant slave ports of all (McEachrane, 2018, p. 476). These global colonial endeavours ran alongside the internal oppression and colonization of the Sami people, the Indigenous people of Northern Scandinavia, fuelled by a growing belief that the White Swede was a member of a superior civilization (McEachrane, 2018, p. 477). All in all, there is simply nothing to suggest that Sweden was actually an exception to European colonial history: it was involved from the start, and along with other Western European nations benefitted directly, and continues to benefit, from slavery and coloniality.

Race biology, race hygiene and eugenics

Parallel to Sweden's hidden colonial history is its pioneering role in race science and eugenics. The Swedish academy were world leaders in the development of race science, and this stemmed from a long tradition of Swedish racial studies. This tradition can be traced back to the 1700s, when Swedish botanist Carl Linnaeus made what is understood to be the first categorization of humans into races in his 1735 work. Although he did not use the term 'race', Linnaeus divided humans into red, white, black and yellow geographically aligned sub-groups, each group bearing a set of fixed behavioural and psychological traits. His work was the foundation for race science. Linnaeus was followed by his compatriot Anders Redzius, who established the cephalic index, a means of establishing race classifications through skull measurements. In the 1870s, the French minister to Sweden was Arthur de Gobineau, the race theorist who developed the theory of an Aryan Master Race. De Gobineau described Swedes as being 'the pure race of the North' and 'the purest branch of the Germanic race' (Biddiss, 1970, p. 225; Broberg & Tydén, 1996, pp. 81–82).

In the immediate post–First World War years, an upholding of the shared belief that Swedes were of a superior race met with a growing fear of degeneration. This fear stemmed from continued mass emigration, a shrinking of the middle class and an increasingly dissatisfied proletariat, and led to publications such as Herman Lundberg's essay, 'The Threat of Degeneration' (1922), in which the author argued, 'The strong increase of the bottom strata forms the most dangerous part of the whole process, for it is their physical and spiritual deficiencies that are such distinct features in their make up'; [yet the] 'racial power of our old farming stock is worth more than its weight in gold' (Lundborg [1922], cited in Broberg & Tydén, 1996, p. 85).

In 1922, the world's first state institute for race biology was founded in Uppsala, charged with the responsibility of preserving Swedish racial stock. Herman Lundborg was the first director, and from the outset the institute had a global impact, inspiring the establishment of Germany's *Kaiser Wilhelm Institut für Rassenhygiene*. The institute's first major task was to measure 100 000 Swedes. The resulting publication, 'The Racial Characters of the Swedish Nation' (Lundborg and Linders, 1926), was printed in English to reach an international audience.

The late 1920s was a time of discussion around the reshaping of Swedish national society, with the introduction of the concept of Sweden as *Folkhemmet*, 'the People's Home'. This was to see a homely society built upon solidarity between classes, and the nation imagined as if it were a family home. Coupled with this cosy notion of national domestication was the beginning of the peak years for Swedish eugenics, with growing public interest in racial and social hygiene projects, and enthusiasm for sterilization programmes targeting marginalized groups to protect the future genetic wellbeing and protect the purity of the white Swedish race (Broberg & Tydén, 1996, p. 83; McEachrane, 2018, p. 478).

Eugenics in practice (1930s–1975)

Sweden's first Sterilization Act was introduced in 1935, with the explicit aim of cleansing the Swedish race of undesirable bodies. The main group targeted for sterilization under the Act was what Broberg and Tydén call, 'the mentally retarded', a category that included people suffering from 'mental illness, feeble-mindedness, or other mental defects', who were forcibly sterilized on a massive scale until the 1950s (Broberg & Tydén, 1996, pp. 102–3).

In 1936, a 'Commission on Population' was set up to discuss expanding the use of forced sterilization as part of social reforms. The Commission's report reflected the nation's commitment to social eugenics: 'Today it is hardly denied by anyone that it is not only justified but also desirable to prevent the procreation of a sick or inferior offspring by means of sterilization' (SOU, 1936, cited in Broberg & Tydén, 1996, p. 106). It went on to argue that the target group for forced sterilizations should be expanded to include 'work-shy individuals, such as prostitutes, vagrants etc.' as well as those people who were, 'psychologically inferior, though not formally legally incompetent, with asocial disposition' (SOU 1936, cited in Broberg & Tydén, 1996, p. 107).

The report led to an updated and expanded Sterilization Act being proposed in Parliament. The ensuing debate certainly indicated the tight alignment of the sterilization programme and race hygiene ideals. For instance, K.G Westman, the Minister of Justice, called the proposed new law 'an important step in the direction of a purification of the Swedish stock, freeing it from the transmission of genetic material which could produce, in future generations, such individuals as are undesirable among a sound and healthy people' (quoted in Broberg & Tydén, 1996, p. 107). His sentiments were echoed by Nils Wohlin of the agrarian party, *Bondeförbundet*, who saw increased forced sterilizations as essential for 'keeping the Swedish stock sound and vigorous for the future', and a number of their fellow parliamentarians, across party lines, pushed for more coercive legislation (Broberg & Tydén, 1996, p. 107).

The result was the passing of the 1941 Sterilization Act. This included further categories of people who could be sterilized without consent: those with severe physical diseases; those with 'an anti-social way of life'; and women – 'for medical reasons'. Almost 3000 people were forcibly sterilized under the 1935 Act, but the 1941 Act saw a huge increase, with 2351 non-consensual sterilizations recorded in the peak year of 1949 alone. From 1950 to 1970, between 1500 and 1700 sterilizations were carried out annually (Broberg & Tydén, 1996, p. 108).[3] The ethnic group that came to be most impacted by the programme were the Tattare (Travellers). Tattare were a racialized group (in that they were classified officially as a race or 'sub-race') who lived on the margins of agrarian societies (Pred, 2000, p. 112). They were assigned set traits: immoral, idle, alcoholic, violent; and described physically as 'dark' and 'Southern looking' (Broberg & Tydén, 1996, p. 125). Some Swedish race scholars, including Herman Lundborg, classified Tattare as the result of mixing between Swedes and Gypsies (Broberg & Tydén, 1996, p. 125). The irregular, transient lives they tended to lead were at odds with the ideals of the new Swedish Welfare State, so the National Board of Social Welfare pushed for regular sterilizations of Tattare women for the reason that 'from a biological and social point of view they are a burden to Swedish society' (1940, cited in Broberg & Tydén, 1996, p. 127). While statistics do not show how many sterilizations were carried out on Tattare, Broberg and Tydén (1996, p. 129), in their extensive studies of Sweden's sterilization history, find many examples of being of Tattare 'stock' or appearance being stated as the reason for sterilization. For example, the reason for sterilization of a teenage girl in 1943 was recorded as: 'Typical *tattare* mentality: evasive, untruthful, and coward'.

Welfare state eugenics was needed to build the 'good Sweden' of the *Folkhem* project, a concept which remains part of a shared Swedish national identity today. Race hygiene ideologies and policies were seen as being required to 'create a sound and healthy people' (Broberg & Tydén, 1996, p. 136). What is imagined as 'good, progressive Sweden' to this day, was built on traditions of race biology and a shared belief in a superior Nordic/Swedish race, and the most extensive sterilization programme imposed on a populace the world has ever seen (Gondouin, 2012). Despite obvious links to German Nazism, Swedish race science and eugenics was not an extreme project of the far right: from the outset it was supported by actors across the political spectrum: Social Democrats, Agrarians, Liberals. In short, Good Sweden was built on racism and eugenic violence, by 'good Swedes'. It would not be unreasonable to argue that the traditions of eugenics underpin the acceptability of the implementation of a herd immunity approach on Swedish society. The idea of sustaining a healthy national body – and economy – by allowing a deadly virus to spread through vulnerable and less valued members of society certainly has very strong echoes of protecting and strengthening Swedish 'racial stock' by sterilizing Other bodies in the nation.

Colour blindness and the good nation

From the late 1960s to the early 2000s Sweden carried out a remarkable transformation in national and global perceptions as it moved from being the world leader in race science and eugenics to being regarded as a progressive, colour blind, anti-racist, anti-colonial nation. A nation where race no longer existed and where visible difference no longer held any meaning. Sweden's racial blindness was part of a broader image of egalitarianism across gender and race lines. The re-imagined, post-racial Swedishness also established the country as the being the 'Third World's benefactor', and the one Western nation standing in solidarity with de-colonization movements worldwide (Hübinette & Lundström, 2014; McEachrane, 2018). McEachrane (2021) describes the reformed Swedish nation as portrayed as a 'moral superpower'.

This move was initiated immediately after the Second World War, when Sweden was involved in drafting the UNESCO Statement on Race (1950), in which the concept of race as a biological truth was dismissed. Key actors in preparing the statement were sociologist Gunnar Myrdal – a robust advocate of eugenic sterilization – and Gunnar Dahlberg, the president of the Institute of Race Biology. The UNESCO Statement led to official rejection of the concept of race in Sweden, and the Institute was renamed *The Department of Medical Genetics* in 1956 (Broberg & Tydén, 1996, pp. 130–1).

Whilst spreading goodness and morality abroad, at home Sweden constructed an extensive welfare state and a Social Democratic political hegemony that dominated the political landscape until the mid-2000s. In a setting where radical social justice and human rights discourses stepped into mainstream politics, Sweden became an officially 'colour-blind state', where the term 'race' became taboo, and was eventually removed from all legislative documents, and the keeping of ethnicity data became prohibited (McEachrane, 2018).

The self-image of globalized goodness meant that Sweden has never reflected upon or reckoned with its racist and colonial history. A colonial power, that was organized around race, *where the very concepts of race and race hygiene originated*, became, almost overnight, the progressive good anti-racist nation with no colonial past. This was despite the fact that the very same actors that developed practical applications of race theory, and endorsed and directed the mass sterilization programme, continued in their positions of knowledge creation. They were, however, now relabelled as *anti-racists*.

Johanna Gondouin (2012) connects Swedish exceptionalism to cultural geographer Katarina Schough's work on the notion of *hyperborean*. Hyperborea is a specifically Nordic version of eurocentrism, which entails the idea of Sweden as being a 'morally and culturally superior and as a peaceful disseminator of culture'. This is how many Swedes relate to colonialism, imagining the Swede as more of a 'participating observer' and an 'impartial explorer in the name of science and culture' than a colonizer (Gondouin, 2012).

This idea of cultural superiority is a means of exonerating Sweden from responsibility for colonialism. The Swede is depicted in colonial discourses as 'the whitest of the white', and thus above the 'racist rating' of colonial hierarchies. The combination of imagined physical and cultural superiority place the hyperborean Swede in an untouchable position: while a (white) participant in the colonial project, the Swede is clearly marked as superior to colonized people, but more importantly the Swede is morally superior to colonizers, and even in a position to criticise the colonial project without being seen – by themselves or others – to be complicit in it (Gondouin, 2012).

Mourning the decline of good white Sweden

Reporting on Sweden and COVID-19 has a theme of the loss of a unique way of being and doing, exemplified by the title of Erik Augustin Palm's article for *The Guardian*, 'Swedish exceptionalism has been ended by coronavirus' (Augustin Palm, 2020). Further adding to this sense of loss is the fact that the Swedish strategy seems to have been praised by the neo-liberal right; the perceived good white nation where social democracy and equality can work is being touted for its neo-liberal emphasis on individual freedoms, its nation-alist tendencies, and even its emphasis on protecting economic interests over human life (Geoghegan, 2021).

I would argue that international fascination with Sweden's COVID-19 response is not just a fascination with the loss of its famed political ideologies and social welfare structures, but is more about Swedish *whiteness*. The interest lies in the fear of the loss of a very unique Swedish whiteness: a whiteness that is pure, the whitest of the white, but also virtuous and *above* racism and colonial exploitation.

Within Sweden, a long, sad decline of good white Sweden has been mourned for some years. Hübinette and Lundstrom (2014) describe Swedish whiteness as being in an era of white melancholia, characterized by a collective longing for an imagined golden era of whiteness. This longed-for era was a time of 'white solidarity', where the white Swede could be good and anti-racist on their own terms. Post-2001 islamophobia and the rise of far-right extremism and the far-right populist party The Sweden Democrats (SD), combined with people of colour voicing their experiences of racism and alienation, has left the nation pining for a mythical time when bodies of colour could be positioned and trusted to behave on white Swedish terms, and when good white Swedes could be good and 'anti-racist' on *their* own terms. This melancholy has been evident from within for some time, yet internationally, evidence of this is a more recent phenomenon.

Concluding reflections

In summary, I have discussed the link between Sweden's COVID-19 response, the international fascination with it and the notion of Swedish exceptionalism. Swedish exceptionalism tends to see Sweden as being a 'globally good' nation, a bastion of human rights, equality and social democracy, that somehow stands outside European histories of Nazism, colonialism and racism. I reflected on how the perception of the Swede as the whitest of the white hyperborean enabled the Swedish subject to be imagined as being above colonial hierarchies, yet this contrasts strongly with a reality of Sweden's leading role in shaping race biology, its role as a colonial nation and its history of eugenicist sterilization programmes targeting unwanted sections of its population. An exploration of Swedish race history indicates that the 'progressive, open' Swedish approach to the virus has much in common with the country's eugenicist past, while an exceptionalist present works to conceal this connection.

External fascination with Sweden's COVID-19 response, I have argued, may go beyond a curiosity about a state doing things differently, to indicate a fixation with and desire for a uniquely Swedish virtuous whiteness. Above all it reflects a fear that this special whiteness is under threat and in decline: it is not just a fascination with white Swedish exceptionalism, but a melancholic lament of its passing.

The hidden history of Swedish race science and eugenics, combined with internationally shared notions of Swedish exceptionalism, could go some way to explaining the possibility of practicing a herd immunity approach to tackling the COVID-19 crisis in the country. While it has been argued that the Swedish approach is based on a unique civic trust where an informed population can be trusted to make the right decisions, a lack of civic knowledge around Sweden's eugenicist history and a belief in Swedish goodness and anti-racism is likely to also have delayed public reflection and resistance. The ideas, implications and ideological backgrounds of herd immunity did not perhaps make for the majority population the immediate connection to a eugenicist history based around 'protecting the pure Swedish stock'. Combined with a nationalistic coming together in defence of international criticism, built around an imagined Swedish way, seen as both a racial behavioural trait and a COVID-19 strategy to suit that trait, this may have restricted internal criticism and further strengthened a collective exceptionalist mentality that saw Sweden as getting it right and the rest of the world as getting it wrong. Indeed, when Anders Tegnell reflected on the Swedish COVID-19 strategy in June 2020, when confronted by criticism from the World Health Organisation and other states, he robustly defended the approach, but made a small concession: 'If we were to encounter the same disease again, knowing exactly what we know about it today, I think we would settle on doing something in between what Sweden did and what the rest of the world has done' (quoted in Habib, 2020). Tegnell's predecessor and mentor Johan Giescke, however, was more outspoken, insisting that 'Sweden is right [and] all the other countries are wrong' (O'Shea, 2020).

Notes

1   Note that people of colour in Swedish discourse tend to be referred to – and classified as – 'immigrants', regardless of immigration status (Lundström, 2017; Wyver, 2021).
2   McEachrane's translation from the original Swedish.
3   These figures only represent the *recorded* operations carried out under the act. Prior to the 1941 act, only sterilizations performed without consent were recorded; Broberg and Tydén (1996, p. 108) point out that sterilizations could always be

carried out voluntarily (that is *with* consent from the patient) on medical grounds, or if there were 'sound reasons of a eugenic, humanitarian or criminological nature'.

References

Anderson, J. (2020). Sweden's Very Different Approach to COVID-19. *Quartz*, 28 April. https://qz.com/1842183/sweden-is-taking-a-very-different-approach-to-covid-19/

Anholt, S. (2021). Good Country Index. https://index.goodcountry.org/

Augustin Palm, E. (2020). 'Swedish Exceptionalism Has Been Ended by Coronavirus'. *The Guardian*, 26 June. https://www.theguardian.com/commentisfree/2020/jun/26/swedish-exceptionalism-coronavirus-covid19-death-toll

Barthes, R. (1993). *Mythologies*. London: Vintage.

Bergsten, S. 2020. Abused and Shunned – Being of Asian Descent in Sweden During Covid-19. *Human Rights Watch*. https://www.hrw.org/news/2020/04/06/abused-and-shunned-being-asian-descent-sweden-during-covid-19

Biddiss, M. D. (1970). *Father of Racist Ideology: The Social and Political Thought of Count Gobineau*. Littlehampton Book Services.

Birrell, I. (2020). COVID 19 Coronavirus: Will Sweden Get the Last Laugh? *New Zealand Herald*, 10 August. https://www.nzherald.co.nz/world/covid-19-coronavirus-will-sweden-get-the-last-laugh/KOBSG5AI373BYGXPMROEX6SG2E/

Bjorklund, K. (2020). The Inside Story of How Sweden Botched Its Coronavirus Response. *Foreign Policy*, 22 December. https://foreignpolicy.com/2020/12/22/sweden-coronavirus-covid-response/#

Broberg, G., & Tydén, M. (1996). Eugenics in Sweden: Efficient Care, edited by G. Broberg & N. Roll-Hansen, 77–149. *Eugenics and the Welfare State: Sterilization Policy in Denmark, Sweden, Norway and Finland*. Michigan State University Press.

Cuthbertson, A. (2020). Coronavirus Tracked: Charting Sweden's Disastrous No-Lockdown Strategy. *The Independent*, 1 June. https://www.independent.co.uk/news/world/europe/coronavirus-lockdown-sweden-death-rate-worst-country-covid-19-a9539206.html

Dagensnyheter. (2020). Professor: 'Inför covid visar sig olikheter och ojämlikhet än mer. *DN.se*, [Professor: In the Face of COVID, Differences and Inequalities Became Even More Visible] 1 July. https://www.dn.se/nyheter/sverige/professor-infor-covid-visar-sig-olikheter-och-ojamlikhet-an-mer/?fbclid=IwAR33Y7XpE2pr9R3sDCYXfqHvyTAHhfHBWlZMoHRtGK5iMSKEPYIckgz1ydY

Daly, M. (2020). Was Sweden Right? Study Suggests Significantly Higher COVID-19 Immunity. *Stuff*, 2 July. https://www.stuff.co.nz/national/health/coronavirus/122011921/coronavirus-was-sweden-right-study-suggests-significantly-higher-covid19-immunity

Geoghegan, P. (2021). Now the Swedish Model Has Failed It's Time to Ask Who Was Pushing It. *The Guardian*, 3 January. https://www.theguardian.com/commentisfree/2021/jan/03/swedish-model-failed-covid-19

Gondouin, J. (2012). Adoption, Surrogacy and Swedish Exceptionalism. *Critical Race and Whiteness Studies*, 8(2), 1–20.

Gustavsson, G. (2020). Has Sweden's Coronavirus Strategy Played into the Hands of Nationalists? *The Guardian*, 1 May. https://www.theguardian.com/world/commentisfree/2020/may/01/sweden-coronavirus-strategy-nationalists-britain

Habib, H. (2020). Has Sweden's Controversial COVID-19 Strategy Been Successful? *BMJ, 369.* doi: https://doi.org/10.1136/bmj.m2376

Hübinette, T., & Lundström, C. (2014). The Three Phases of Hegemonic Whiteness: Understanding Racial Temporalities in Sweden. *Social Identities: Journal for the Study of Race, Nation and Culture, 20*(6), 423–37.

Hübinette, T., & Sjöblom, L. (2015). Det räcker med 'gulinghumor' nu SVT' [That's Enough with 'Yellow Humour' Now SVT]. *Expressen,* 2 June. https://www.expressen .se/debatt/det-racker-med-gulinghumor-nu-svt/

Jackson, R. (2020). Has Sweden Made a Fatal Mistake with COVID-19 Coronavirus? *New Zealand Herald,* 28 May. https://www.nzherald.co.nz/nz/rod -jackson-has-sweden-made-a-fatal-mistake-with-covid-19-coronavirus/RUR7CV376 CXFC4Q2M7J7YAYW6M/

The Local. (2020). We Experienced a Racist Assault for Wearing Facemasks. 20 May. https://www.thelocal.se/20200520/we-experienced-a-racist-assault-for-wearing-face -masks

Lundborg, H. & Linders, F.J. (1926). *The Racial Characters of the Swedish Nation: Anthropologia Suecia MCMXXVI.* Almqvist & Wiksell.

Lundström, C. (2017). The White Side of Migration: Reflections on Race, Citizenship and Belonging in Sweden. *Nordic Journal of Migration Research, 7*(2), 79–87.

McEachrane, M. (2018). Universal Human Rights and the Coloniality of Race in Sweden. *Human Rights Review, 19,* 471–93.

McEachrane, M. (2021). Will European Countries Ever Take Meaningful Steps to End Colonial Legacies? *The Conversation,* 22 February. https://theconversation .com/will-european-countries-ever-take-meaningful-steps-to-end-colonial-legacies -148581

Karlsson, J.J. (2020). Sofia, 19, spelade in rasismen hon utsätts för: 'folk tror inte på det'. [Sofia, 19, Recorded the Racism She Was the Victim of Because 'People Don't Believe It'] *SVT,* 28 December. https://www.svt.se/nyheter/inrikes/sofia-spelade-in-rasismen -hon-fick-motta-pa-chattforum-polisanmaldes?fbclid=IwAR0sFE5GyzfWsbDGIkjL jOkvgiDoAojdlEHeAdJhTUKaDC51HtptnBKDi9w

O'Shea, P. (2020). Sweden and Japan Are Paying the Price for COVID Exceptionalism. *The Conversation,* 18 December. https://theconversation.com /sweden-and-japan-are-paying-the-price-for-covid-exceptionalism-151974

Pred, A. (2000). *Even in Sweden: Racisms, Racialized Spaces, and the Popular Geographical Imagination.* University of California Press.

Rothschild, N. (2020). The Hidden Flaw in Sweden's Anti-Lockdown Strategy. *Foreign Policy,* 21 April. https://foreignpolicy.com/2020/04/21/sweden-coronavirus -anti-lockdown-immigrants/

Siret, M. (2016). Sweden Officially 'Goodest' Country in the World, Study Says. *Independent,* 2 June. https://www.independent.co.uk/news/world/politics/sweden -goodest-country-world-good-country-index-a7061341.html

Worldometers. (2021). Coronavirus Cases. October 4. https://www.worldometers.info /covid

Wyver, R. (2015). Swedish Asians Call for an End to 'Gook Humour'. *Kultwatch,* 8 June. https://kultwatch.se/2015/06/08/swedish-asians-call-for-an-end-to-gook-humour/

Wyver, R. (2020). From Flat-Packed Furniture to Fascism: Exploring the Role of the Transracial Adoptee in Fantasies of Swedish Goodness. *Interventions: International Journal of Postcolonial Studies, 22*(7), 897–915.

Wyver, R. (2021). Too Brown to Be Swedish, too Swedish to Be Anything Else: Mimicry and Menace in Swedish Transracial Adoption Narratives. *Social Identities: Journal for the Study of Race, Nation and Culture, 27*(3), 394–409.

5   Time back! A research manifesto for Indigenous urgencies

Simon Lambert

Introduction

In the first few months of the COVID-19 pandemic, state and non-state authorities scrambled to respond to the rapidly escalating crisis. On 23 April 2020, the Canadian federal government launched a COVID-19 Immunity Task Force (CITF) 'charged with leading a Canada-wide effort to help determine the extent of severe acute respiratory syndrome (SARS) CoV-2 infection in Canada (in the general population as well as in specific communities and priority populations)' (COVID 19 Immunity Task Force, 2020). In fulfilling this mandate, the CITF was to invest CAN\$9.2 million in a 'comprehensive nationwide Indigenous seroprevalence study, which has at its heart the respectful engagement of First Nations, Inuit and Métis communities across Canada' (ibid.). Seroprevalence describes the number or percentage of people in a population who test positive for a particular disease, based on blood serum (serology) specimens. Key collaborators for this research were sought from a Canadian Institutes of Health Research (CIHR) funded Network Environments for Indigenous Health Research (NEIHR) Program, comprising nine networks across Canada (Canadian Institutes of Health Research, 2021a). The data that was to be collected was intended to 'help guide public health measures in Indigenous communities to prevent the transmission of SARS CoV-2 as well as to help identify health services needed to care for Indigenous Peoples with COVID-19 across Canada'. The proposal was titled 'The Indigenous Journeys through COVID-19: A National Indigenous Seroprevalence Cross-Sectional and Community Sentinel Cohort Study', or 'Indigenous Journeys' for short.

Eight months later, at the 2020 Annual General Assembly of the Assembly of First Nations (AFN), one of the 22 resolutions moved and passed by the gathered Chiefs (representing 634 First Nations across Canada with over

900 000 members) sought a moratorium on 'Indigenous Journeys' (Assembly of First Nations, 2020, p. 9). A communication from the Nominated Principal Investigator (NPI) announced the suspension of the project, ironically on the same day that it was reported that the seroprevalence approach was not providing the data initially envisaged by its proponents (Ling, 2021).

From its initial launch to its final demise, the strategies and tactics deployed by participants of the proposed seroprevalence project reveal a pattern of chaos recognizable to any student of emergency law. Legal and methodological approaches in the face of an emergency or disaster require an understanding of the conditions under which actors have the authority to deviate from accepted norms, in which jurisdictions and for how long. This chapter uses the failure of the Indigenous seroprevalence project as an illustration of the obligations and pathways required of an Indigenous disaster research manifesto (the following chapter by Dittmer and Lorenz is also devoted to disaster). By examining the array of opportunities and challenges that arose from the declaration of the pandemic, through the formulation of research funding calls, to the design of programs and projects, the theoretical and practical implications of specifically Indigenous research can be described.

Indigenous emergencies as spatial and temporal dislocation: modernity as urgency

While some have labelled modern society itself as a world of unintended risk (for example Beck, 1992), Indigenous experiences of colonization trump any academic ascriptions of collective accidental 'disaster'. Across Indigenous and non-Indigenous scholarship, we see the systematic stripping of Indigenous security and safety (Daschuk, 2013; Dunbar-Ortiz, 2014; United Nations, 2007). From the Papal Bulls of the fifteenth century (Vera, 2012) to the explicit oppression and violence of the twentieth and early twenty-first centuries (OHCHR/Secretariat of the Permanent Forum on Indigenous Issues, 2017; Truth and Reconciliation Commission, 2016), Indigenous Peoples have been excluded, denied, erased and exploited by imperial, colonial and now, neoliberal forces. While we can draw a direct line between the enclosures of European commonwealth societies and patterns of imposition forced on Indigenous communities, colonization imposes on Indigenous Peoples an oppressive regime of wealth extraction and risk creation. To understand this better, I draw on Loevy (2016) and her re-interpretation of modern emergency laws as a critical lens through which to view Indigenous health research strategies in times of disaster.

Loevy (2016) provides a challenge to disaster studies scholars in her disman-
tling of a dichotomy between, on the one hand, the normal functioning of a
society, and on the other, an event or issue that requires the suspension of
rights and freedoms to protect or preserve that society. Arguing that what
appear as urgent decisions in response to immediate events are really implemented with a view to framing a future *post*-disaster landscape, Loevy uses a
Žižekian tool to present the almost mythical (for the United States) figure of
Lincoln in a movie scene. In Spielberg's (2012) *Lincoln*, Lincoln (played by
Englishman Daniel Day Lewis) delays the ending of the brutal Civil War to
force the passing of the abolition amendment before the war powers invested
in him are revoked by peace (Loevy, 2016, p. 1). During the US-led 'war on
terror' the White House had a similar fear of peace threatening the future of the
United States and pursued 'get out of jail cards' in the event a post-emergency
legislative assembly sought to examine the actions of officials involved in ren-
dition, torture and killing.[1] Loevy's (2016, p. 4) point is that emergencies are no
longer unexpected or exceptional events: 'normal times have been replaced by
a constant state of exception'. The US authorities shaped a post-war socio-legal
framework to facilitate a permanent war. From an Indigenous perspective, this
is the standard operating procedure for oppressive state regimes.

Disaster studies are similarly hampered by a dichotomous arrangement distinguishing stability and assumptions of a 'normal' environment from moments
of sudden rupture. Emergency management is deployed in response to the
sudden occurrence of an event, often 'unprecedented', at least to the majority
of citizens and news consumers. Disasters are interpreted as temporally and
spatially discrete events, before and after which stable and safe society is the
norm (Hewitt, 1983). Indigenous scholarship is ideally situated to critique
emergency laws and their role in causing and resolving urgency.

From First Contact, Indigenous communities confronted exceptional circumstances, radical deviations from Indigenous norms (Ewen, 1994; O'Malley,
2012; Shannon, 2008). However, it is important to remember that, as comprehensive as colonization has been, the effects were neither universal nor
uniform across Indigenous worlds as recorded by Indigenous orally transmitted accounts of newcomers, their new ways and their impacts (Nabokov,
1999). Although Indigenous scholarship has re-interpreted Indigenous endurance through these momentous experiences as 'resilience' (Lambert, 2014), as
Penehira et al. (2014) argue, the approach is best described as one of constant
resistance.

In this chapter, I seek to support efforts that will simultaneously slow the
frantic nature of decision making that Indigenous communities face, and

speed up the empowerment of Indigenous Peoples in addressing Disaster Risk Reduction (DRR). I will structure the argument using Loevy's categorization of four domains through which emergency powers operate, namely (1) the defined conditions that (2) allow for deviations from norms (3) over a given jurisdiction (4) for a limited time.[2] While this typology hints at a possibility of strengthening the theoretical understanding of disasters and emergencies, what Lovey draws attention to is the contingency of emergency law, and the many choices available in its operationalization.

My thinking on Indigenous emergency management, and health crises in particular, has been very much shaped by several years in Saskatchewan, Canada, Treaty Six territory and the Homeland of the Métis. While health care was deliberated in the many Treaty discussions that took place across Turtle Island, only in Treaty Six (in 1876) is there explicit reference made to a 'medicine chest' (Lux, 2018). Yet Indigenous People across Treaty Six (and beyond) experience appalling health (Tait et al., 2013). What Indigenous Peoples faced with COVID-19 had a very long and tragic prequel.

With this long history in mind, I now return to the Public Health Agency of Canada (PHAC) seroprevalence study titled 'Indigenous Journeys through COVID-19: Development of a National Indigenous Seroprevalence Cohort study' (hereafter 'Indigenous Journeys') to examine: how the Indigenous emergency was defined; what authorities were allowed or expected to transgress normal operating procedures; what jurisdictions were involved; and the temporal characteristics of the emergency. The purpose is to appreciate the manipulation of time and space to effect research strategies that purport to benefit Indigenous communities.

Indigenous journeys: the seroprevalence proposal

As a medical technique and pandemic response, seroprevalence sits within the wider Canadian context of Indigenous health and wellbeing. While countless shocking events detail the realities of Indigenous health in Canada, just one will serve to illustrate the racist reality. In 2020, Joyce Echaquan, of Atikamekw Nation in southwestern Quebec, Canada, was subject to racist slurs by hospital staff before her death (Godin, 2020). Echaquan managed to live stream the insults as proof of something that is well known among Indigenous People (Turpel-Lafond, 2020), but still presents as a somehow fresh scandal. Joyce Echaquan should not have had to be resilient to the level of hatred directed towards her. Positioning resilience as an admirable callus on our collective lives, acquired over generations of oppression, risks reifying the status quo of vulnerability and diverts attention from a key component of resilience to disaster, namely sovereignty.

The structural racism of states like Canada has embedded vulnerabilities leading to vastly different death rates. The 2009 swine flu pandemic – caused by the H1N1 virus – provided an important indication of how future pandemics could unfold. Statistics Canada recorded about 4 percent of the population identifying as Indigenous, yet Indigenous People[3] accounted for over 17 percent of reported H1N1 deaths during the first wave and almost 9 percent of deaths during the second wave (Helferty et al., 2010). Over 25 percent of critically ill patients from 39 Intensive Care Units in the first wave (Kumar et al., 2009) and over 20 percent of patients from 12 pediatric ICUs (both waves combined) were Indigenous (Tran et al., 2012). Of all reported pregnant cases, 18 percent were Indigenous women (Rolland-Harris et al., 2012). While there were significant knowledge gaps (National Collaborating Centre for Aboriginal Health, 2016), it was clear that Indigenous Peoples across Canada experienced more severe impacts from the virus.

Seroprevalence studies were to be a key source of data in the Canadian government's responses to COVID-19 (Lai et al., 2020), with an Indigenous component built into them. The 'Investment Note' for the Indigenous Journeys study was developed and approved in July 2020, and an Indigenous NPI engaged by PHAC to negotiate the contract was approved on 12 August (PHAC, 2020). An Indigenous Advisory Circle (IAC) was established to

> provide advice and guidance to this Indigenous COVID-19 seroprevalence and immunity study as well as to other studies supported by the Task Force that have Indigenous aspects. The IAC included representation from First Nations, Métis and Inuit communities, Universities, and organizations, and academia, while ensuring language, gender, and geographical diversity. It also includes Elders/Knowledge Keepers.

The overwhelming majority of IAC members were Indigenous, a point that I will return to in the discussion.

A press release (circulated but never released) repeated the basic methodological approach, and the role of the NEIHRs, with the Chair noting,

> One of our top guiding principles is respecting First Nations, Inuit and Métis Peoples' right to self-determination by supporting health research based on scientific

excellence and community partnerships. It is imperative that Indigenous communities involved feel they have a place at the table, which they have not had previously, and that the findings are fully shared with each community.

The primary objectives were to:

(1) determine the prevalence of COVID-19 antibodies in First Nations, Métis, and Inuit communities;
(2) understand the social determinants of infection, symptoms, severity and outcomes in these communities;
(3) explore using health services data linkage where possible to assess Indigenous population patterns in COVID-19 health care use, complications and outcomes using administrative health data;
(4) collaborate with international Indigenous networks and the World Health Organization (WHO) to develop international studies with other Indigenous communities worldwide.

The intent of 'Indigenous Journeys' was that '. . . a national cross-sectional cohort will be established by sampling blood spot tests from ≈6,000 household sites, resulting in a total sample size of ≈18,000. Within each household, three samples will be used to represent a child/youth, an adult, and an Elder'. The serum itself was to be self-sampled by a technique called 'dried blood spot' test that 'can be performed in the comfort of one's home by taking drops of blood from a finger using a spring-loaded lancet . . . and placing it onto an absorbent filter paper' (COVID 19 Immunity Task Force, 2021). Once this filter paper is dry, the test is sealed and 'shipped to a lab at ambient temperature through regular carrier services'. Once in the laboratory, the samples are tested for the presence of COVID-19 antibodies. Phase 2 was to maintain the initial cohort and continue with three monthly samplings.

Several online meetings of the IAC took place from May to September, coinciding with teleconferences between the NPI, Indigenous government officials and staff and NPIs of the nine NEIHRs. Several of the NEIHRs meetings were contentious as the proposal was framed as necessary and urgent, with community lives at stake, yet several representatives questioned the management of the project. Commitment from potential collaborators and partners was unclear with a key collaborator (First Nations Information Governance Centre) withdrawing.

Numerous issues were not resolved during the meetings and follow-up communications. Notwithstanding the difficulties in engaging with Indigenous communities during a pandemic (physical visits from researchers being forbidden by institutional ethics processes), the storage and ownership of blood samples, and subsequent use of these samples, was particularly challenging (for further discussion of COVID-19 and ethical issues, see Dare & Kingsbury in this volume). The final circulated proposal noted, '[t]he core content of the study that will be consistent across all sampling sites will be reviewed by the PHAC Research Ethics Board. Ethics approval for the core data will done by PHAC, however, each NEIHR [sic] will obtain ethical review and approvals needed for any region-specific research design'. This regionally tailored approach was undermined by the Contribution Agreement that stated:

(1) S16.1 Any intellectual property that arises out of or under this Agreement shall be owned by the Recipient or by a third party, as set out in an agreement between the Recipient and such third party. The Recipient shall report to Canada what Materials, if any, have been created or developed under this Agreement.
(2) S16.2 Canada will review the list of Materials provided by the Recipient pursuant to section 16.1 for the purpose of determining if Canada wishes to negotiate a license agreement, separate from this Agreement, for the rights to have and to use any such Materials.

Examining the government's announcements, seroprevalence proposal drafts, including the Contribution Agreement, planned research structures and the AFN Resolution 4, we see the four domains of the Manin/Loevy typology in play. First, the *conditions* of the emergency were framed by the rapidly escalating pandemic whose spread was massively facilitated by the extensive international travel that many people engage in, whether for business, leisure or family reasons. The urgency of rising infections, hospital admissions and deaths saw disruption cascading through highly devolved supply chains, associated precarious employment and often exacerbated by poor housing and transport options for many 'key workers' (Franco, 2020). The impacts are, of course, gendered, with women disproportionately taking on extra tasks while losing their livelihoods at faster rates than men (Seck et al., 2021). Indigenous communities in Canada were flagged as being more vulnerable (Arriagada et al., 2020), reiterating the already existing disaster of colonization.

The *authority* involved was comprised of federal and provincial health agencies, which in many instances includes Indigenous organizations, although their roles are often circumscribed by structural inequities. Health, as noted by the Canadian Supreme Court, 'is not a matter which is subject to specific constitutional assignment but instead is *an amorphous topic* (emphasis added) which can be addressed by valid federal or provincial legislation, depending in the circumstances of each case on the nature or scope of the health problem in question'.[4] Butler and Tiedeman (2011, p. 1) note that '[i]t is not surprising, given the period in which it was written, that the Constitution Act, 1867 does not explicitly include 'health' as a legislative power assigned either to Parliament . . . or to the provincial legislatures'. There is a parallel in Treaty discourse with the 'medicine chest' listed in Treaty Six no longer sufficient to encompass modern health care.

Without dismissing the importance of jurisdiction, I think it only fair to warn readers that the jurisdictions involved in Indigenous worlds are juxtaposed across time and space and are highly contested to the point of violent resistance, and even more violent oppression by state and corporate forces. There is, of course, continuous and contested positions within Indigenous groups. Aspects of this internal, endogenous, dynamism can also be discerned within the 'Indigenous Journeys' proposal. Yet it is colonial discourse, designed to dispossess, dilute and diminish Indigenous control, that dominates the COVID-19 landscape and as the (Western scientific) health data shows, colonial authorities have been devastatingly effective.

The *temporal* characteristics of this emergency are what interest me most, and where I see the most challenging research *management* issues. Management? Surely I mean a methodological snap, a remedial step or intellectual leap? I will return to this theme in the discussion but wish to alert readers to the question of 'What would *you* do?' if faced with the urgencies of an Indigenous response to a pandemic?

Case study: seroprevalence as a temporary front

From one perspective, the failure of the seroprevalence proposal can be explained by the lack of necessary relationships sufficient for any research proposals, let alone one that self-declares an Indigenous journey. Relationality is culturally and methodologically central to Indigenous approaches, participants were geographically scattered, unable to meet face to face and many were busy supporting their own Indigenous health networks while maintaining households, supporting parents and siblings, homeschooling their children and so on (for an extended discussion of care see Huppatz and Craig in this collection). However, through an emergency law lens we can detect patterns and a level of – for want of a better term – predictability. This is not to say the decisions of participants can be known before they are made but that the parameters within which those decisions are made can be drawn.

The conditions: what is the emergency?

The conditions for COVID-19 extended, indeed began, beyond the Canadian border as the pandemic was officially declared by the WHO on 30 January 2020[5] (World Health Organization, 2021). Suspected origins for this virus include a Chinese 'wet market', bat caves (also in China), with the increasing contact between human activities, including intensive stock rearing, and previously isolated ecosystems also pointed to as providing the ideal conditions for inter-species jumps (Wallace and Wallace offer an extended discussion of the production of pandemics in their chapter).

Wider socio-political forces further frame these emergency conditions. Public discourse was comprised of the dynamic interplay of political leaders, senior health officials, epidemiologists, lobbyists and many 'influencers' who promulgated views, interpretations and strategies, often via social media. Diplomatic tensions were revealed in the variance of state responses, enflamed by accusations of accidental or deliberate releases of the virus and multiple conspiracies that, as is often the case, ranged from the feasible (bumbling government officials and opaque Chinese statements) to the fantastical (a US tech billionaire was implanting chips into people via vaccines). Previous health emergencies have exposed the difficulties of achieving a consensus for appropriate responses when there is inconsistency between public health messaging and comments or platforms of individuals or groups (World Health Organization, 2005). The ease with which media personalities, political or business leaders and momentary social media stars undermined urgent health campaigns has made it difficult for the health sector to implement a key precondition of public preventive behavior, that is, communicate that such action is needed, is perhaps one of history's more remarkable inverses of a disruptive technological innovation.

Six weeks passed before the Canadian Prime Minister announced restrictions on entry to Canada (16 March) to be implemented shortly after midnight Eastern Time, 18 March. Entry was to be restricted to US and Canadian citizens and permanent residents and families, as well as flight crew members who did not display symptoms (Harris, 2020). Three weeks after that, the Royal Canadian Mounted Police had confirmed they were tasked with enforcing the 2005 Quarantine Act (ibid.),[6] enacted after the 2003 SARS epidemic. As business leaders sought financial support, many workers were laid off or suspended, and the rapid collapse of supply chains saw large increases in unemployment in a 'gravely wounded' world economy (United Nations Conference on Trade and Development, 2020; see McDonagh in this collection for discussion of the global economy).

In the first weeks of the emergency, clearly global from its initial conditions, Indigenous Peoples watched with considerable anxiety. As noted, in Canada Indigenous communities were disproportionately impacted by SARS, and little had been achieved in the intervening years to reduce their vulnerability to infectious diseases. Poor quality housing, overcrowding, limited primary health services, poverty and racism (Turpel-Lafond, 2020) continued to undermine Indigenous efforts at development and self-determination. The social determinants of health for Indigenous Peoples in Canada 'reflects the socioeconomic, environmental, and political contexts of their lives, a context inextricable from past and contemporary colonialism' (Greenwood et al., 2018, p. 1646). While the final COVID-19 story has yet to be told, Indigenous leaders knew their communities were vulnerable.

This collective insight of Indigenous vulnerability is a product of the post-disaster landscape on which many if not most Indigenous communities survive. Indigenous worlds are a result of disaster risk creation (Lambert, 2022). The consequent vulnerabilities to, among other infectious diseases, COVID-19, echoes the exposure of Indigenous People to other risks and hazards that are arguably emergencies for those Indigenous communities facing those conditions. Saskatchewan doctors specializing in HIV treatment wrote an open letter to the Saskatchewan Provincial government, stating 'whether the provincial government chooses to recognize it or not, we are in a state of emergency with a deadly infectious disease' (Vogel, 2016, p. 1071). Their fears over the risks of HIV are matched by disastrous expansion of opioid availability (Russell et al., 2016), horrific suicide statistics (Tait et al., 2017) and missing and murdered Indigenous People (National Inquiry into Missing and Murdered Indigenous Women and Girls, 2019), which all reflect an ongoing disaster that threatens to have no end.

Yet the Saskatchewan provincial government was under no legal requirement to initiate an emergency response to the request from medical professionals. Indeed, they and other governments (provincial/territorial and federal) have systematically ignored declarations of emergencies by Indigenous leaders over suicide (James, 2019), lack of potable water (Eabametoong First Nation, 2019; Nunn, 2018) and resource conflicts (Roache & Moore, 2020). The conditions of impoverishment, ill health, poor educational outcomes and unemployment that pervade Indigenous communities are an outcome of colonization and would require decolonization for an effective response. With that, and looking to the second component of emergency law, what authorities are vested with the powers to 'deviate from the norm'?

The authorities: who is in control?

Sovereign is he who decides on the exception.[7] (Carl Schmitt)

The Loevy–Marin model of modern emergency powers assumes these powers are not static or inert. Instead, the response/recovery nexus of any crisis is contingent on whose interests are identified and addressed as being at risk, and for colonized peoples this authority is primarily wielded by a colonial master who was rarely liable for the loss of Indigenous lives or assets.[8] Loevy recounts an example from colonial operations in India in the case of *Bhagat Singh and Others vs. The King Emperor* (Loevy, 2016, pp. 70–72). Singh was an Indian nationalist charged with killing a British officer and subsequently convicted by a special tribunal convened by the Governor-General under his emergency powers. He appealed to the Privy Council on the grounds that there was no emergency. The appeal was dismissed on the reasoning that the indefinability of an emergency was resolved by accepting 'it has to be judged by someone' (Loevy, 2016, p. 71). The person or position that would address any and all emergencies was the Governor-General. A key insight we can take from Loevy's work for Indigenous discourse is that while emergency powers enable the 'authorities' to return society to 'normality' – with force if necessary – this normality itself is unexamined.

The interpretation of emergency powers as being contingent does not dismiss the hierarchy deployed in Canadian emergency management. This structure, recognizable across the international emergency arena, sees Federal/Provincial/Territorial (FPT) Ministers occupying the top tier, with FPT Deputy Ministers in the second tier, senior officials in a third tier (Public Safety Canada, 2017, p. 15) and so on down to emergency responders. However, globally, the pandemic saw a dominant role played by health authorities and *not* disaster organizations. In Canada, the Constitution Act, 1867 gave provinces the authority to establish and operate hospitals, asylums and charities; the federal government had jurisdiction over marine hospitals and quarantine.[9]

A key authority in the COVID-19 response is the PHAC. PHAC was established in the aftermath of the 2003 SARS epidemic as a Legislated Service Agency (Tiedeman, 2006). Among other funding, PHAC administered the Safe Restart Agreement (SRA), a federal investment of CAN$19 billion to support provinces and territories to 'safely restart their economies and make our country more resilient to possible future surges in cases of COVID-19'. The funding was to support testing and contract tracing, a recognized approach to minimize risk of community spread.[10]

Yet serious concerns were raised by the media on the level of preparedness the agency, and by default, the country, had for a pandemic. Several months after the declaration of a pandemic, reports revealed the Global Public Health Intelligence Network (established and maintained by Canada) was severely under resourced. In addition, the key position of chief health surveillance officer was vacant since 2017 and was evidently due to be eliminated (Public Health Agency of Canada, 2021, p. 10). The key state authority in a pandemic response seemed somewhat underprepared.

Despite the escalating emergency – the federal government had released modeling that indicated up to 300 000 Canadians could die from COVID-19 (Public Health Agency of Canada, 2020) – the Prime Minister said that he was not planning to invoke the sweeping Emergencies Act, which would allow federal authorities to assume powers normally reserved for provinces and territories.[11] Towards the end of 2021, the Scientific Director of the Institute of Indigenous Peoples Health (IIPH) was exposed as a 'pretendian', someone who has faked their Indigenous positionality (Leo, 2021). While not the only instance, the fact that this was the most senior 'Indigenous' health researcher in Canada further shook Indigenous Peoples' trust in the authorities.

This shocking case of identity fraud draws attention to the dominance of federal, provincial and territorial structures over Indigenous governance structures. Indigenous politics are a combination of traditional and colonial practices. For the purposes of this chapter, readers need to maintain their awareness of, on the one hand, the prevailing racism of the current political–economic regime and, on the other, the variance of opinion, fears, vulnerability and aspirations within communities. In one widely reported case, a former chief condemned the rollout of the Moderna vaccine in his community. This community of 4000 was selected as one of the first to be vaccinated in that province because of its large population and proximity to so-called red zones (COVID-19 hotspots), and because it was the location of an elders' long-term care facility. In his words, the community were like 'experimental rats of this experimental vaccine' (Pashagumskum, 2021). However, the *current* chief of that nation stated he and his family would get the vaccine when it comes to his community. 'Generally speaking, people are coming out now getting the facts about the vaccine and are participating'. While the legacies leading to vaccine hesitancy in Indigenous communities are profound, many leaders and community members freely, even eagerly, seek the latest that medical science can offer them. Yet, as the flimsiness of IIPH's – and therefore federal – authority was revealed by academic fakery, Indigenous vulnerabilities to state and state agents remains.

Of course, Indigenous Peoples and Indigenous Knowledges (IK) can and should inform localized emergency response (Lambert & Scott, 2019). Space precludes an extensive discussion of IK; for the purposes of this review, it is interpreted as nothing more (but nothing less) than the knowledge held by Indigenous collectives regardless of source, character, medium or mode. This is perhaps too broad a church for some Indigenous scholars. For the purposes of my argument, the key characteristics of IK in emergencies (Lambert & Mark-Shadbolt, 2021) are: (1) insight and experiences of relevant hazards, risks and vulnerabilities, as well as resources, strengths and local intelligence; (2) ethical and safe approaches, attribution, ownership, use and transmission; (3) a curiosity and processes to learn more; and (4) the reassertion of sovereignty over the relevant data by the Peoples in whose jurisdiction the emergency is bounded or present.

I will not over-emphasize the insights, diversity and complexity of IK. Rather, I argue that the public sphere from which legal powers emerge is a 'marketplace of ideas [with] entrenched power structures [and] ideologies' (Ingber, 1984, pp. 85–86). As Bhagat Singh and Others found out in their challenge to the King Emperor, the power to assert what is *correct* enables judgements on what is *right*. Indigenous institutions, with their origins in their own knowledges and values, are positioned as *wrong*, and therefore illegitimate.

The jurisdictions: where are the borders?

How can we draw a boundary around an emergency? The transnational aspect of disasters is now well known, exemplified by global heating and climate change. What are the implications of borders (real and imagined) in a pandemic, given that Indigenous communities are subjected to illegitimate borders? The Saskatchewan Provincial Archives hold a series of reports on wildfire and Indian 'reservations'.[12] These reports contain the names and number of people employed to fight fires, their supplies, which jurisdictions were involved and where blame and therefore fiscal responsibility lay. For example, in a report on a fire at Pelican Lake, 17 May 1942, the Director of Indian Affairs Branch argued that as the fire originated beyond the local reserve, and on Crown lands, the cost of containment ($70.50) was chargeable to the Forest Service, 'in the same manner as, on previous occasions, the cost for fighting fires spreading from Indian Reserves to outside lands has been billed to our Service'.[13]

The mention of wildfires is deliberate. Identifying responsibility to the transnational phenomenon of wildfires (and their attendant impact on air quality) is a pressing concern. Indigenous communities are disproportionately impacted by wildfires and floods, with on-reserve households evacuated at 18 times the rate of those off reserve (Kuiack, 2018). Audra Simpson's (2008) examination of Canadian accusations of smuggling against Iroquois tobacco merchants exposes an interesting fallacy of colonial sovereignty, namely that everyone else thinks these claims are legitimate.

Of course, US violence against Indigenous Peoples south of the 49th parallel is likewise horrific, misplaced and proceeds as racist colonial structures were intended. Addressing the causal conditions of global heating, as with COVID-19, is impossible without multinational collaboration, and possibly impossible even with collective global endeavors. When Indigenous People suffer, the system is not broken but merely functioning as it was intended (Razack, 2015). Indigenous communities have had their sovereign status, including the right to identify and manage their own emergencies, systematically and violently taken from them. Recent calls for 'Land back' demand the return of Indigenous lands, waters and resources to Indigenous Peoples and their communities. Their riskscapes are beyond their control and many times beyond their knowledge, although by that I mean what community can be expected to know how to manufacture modern vaccines? Access to the necessary health care, including medicines, therapies, surgical techniques, organ donation and transplants and so on, is what a medicine chest translates to in the time of COVID-19. My use of 'time back' in my title is designed to highlight the temporal aspect of, in this case, a health crisis in which Indigenous communities are responding to ongoing events as their experiences continue to highlight health inequities. The time to embed 'resilience' to this latest pandemic has passed.

The time: when is this all over?

I recall an interview with a Māori Elder who, when asked why European diplomacy with Māori so often failed, tapped his wrist in the universal (but completely modern) sign for 'time'. Gregg and Kneese (2019, n.p.) position *timed* time, the clock in their example, as a social technology that authorizes 'a singular source to propel collective activity'. The precedents for the contraction of time can be traced in the workplace clock (Gregg & Kneese, 2019), the air raid siren, Cold War immanent mutual assured destruction, the 'Limits to Growth' (Meadows & Meadows, 2007) and modern financial transactions in which milliseconds separate electronic trades for the arbitrage of cents (Lanchester, 2018).

As the timeframes for failure have drastically shortened on local, regional and global scales, Indigenous Peoples may ironically be strengthened through Western needs to understand and reduce exposure to cascading disaster risks. This is observed through Indigenous fire management that sits within wider issues of self-determination for Indigenous communities of their lands, waters and biological heritage. Despite Western sciences finding that IK was accurate (and therefore Indigenous practices insightful), modern legislation and environmental management policies primarily defaulted to prevention and suppression instead of the mitigation of fire hazard through what can only be described as a more intelligent approach towards the manipulation of ecosystems, including prescribed burns. Many Indigenous Peoples continue a remarkable panoply of practices whose value is more apparent as the legacy of colonial models of fire management continue to fail around the world. Admittedly, there is very little preventing PHAC in continuing their sero-prevalence strategy but Indigenous sovereignty was explicitly displayed by Indigenous governance structures as they 'call time' to assert their primacy in research 'on' their communities.

Are we becoming ever more urgent? That colonization is the defining experience of indigeneity is reinforced by constant demand for decolonizing oppressive structures.

Discussion

Despite the growing research literature, government and Non-Governmental Organization reports, shocking headlines and plaintive pleas for support in the Indigenous world, reduction in Indigenous disaster risks seem rare to the point of obscurity. Drawing solely on Indigenous experiences of pandemics we can see the same gamut of fear, violence, physical separation, resignation, strategic resistance and renaissance. In the disaster and emergency field (diverse and atheoretical as it is; see Alexander, 2017), the dominant approach remains in thrall to an obviously discredited school of calamity that saw disasters as rare and unpredictable events, a technocratic challenge that is amenable to prediction and control, with no intent or perceived need for wider understanding of what is happening (Hewitt, 1983). Despite the clear shift in thinking signaled by the UN Sendai Framework for Disaster Risk Reduction that sees the source of risk as endogenous to society instead of exogenous, top-down responses controlled or influenced by political–economic interests entrench mal-development that embeds future risks to pre-existing and cascading hazards.[14]

The Manin/Loevy model of emergencies, and their response, as being contingent is in accord with Indigenous experiences. These experiences frame colonization as the uber-disaster, and that I argue all Indigenous Peoples are still responding to, and still recovering from (Lambert, 2022). This does position Indigenous communities as vulnerable by default, hardly an optimistic start in addressing DRR, although by default I mean that the succession of imperial, colonial and neoliberal forces have *violently* deposed Indigenous sovereignty and built on the Western foundation of Schmittian legal theory that enforced a *non*-Indigenous constitutional right 'to decide on the exception'. But First Contact with Europeans was not necessarily an emergency for Indigenous Peoples who oftentimes rescued famished and imperiled explorers and settlers (Nabokov, 1999).[15] It has been an emergency ever since. As N'de (Apache) scholar Mario Villa says, 'we are in the same fkn room as serial killers. Our Peoples need to manage this' (personal communication). Again and again, the risk profile of Indigenous Peoples is entwined with socio-economic conditions (or whatever combination of domains can be conjured) that are imposed by usurping nations. Hewitt (1983, p. 10, emphasis in the original) draws an interesting parallel between calamity and Foucault's critique of madness in that both ascriptions of disorder challenge hegemonic notions of order. Western management of 'insanity' and 'calamity' see a 'careful, pragmatic and disarming *placement* of the problem'. The reserve and pass systems of the Canadian colonial state can be seen from this perspective as the deliberate dis/re-location of Indigenous communities, often on to more hazardous landscapes. The modern history of violence faced by First Nations, Métis and Inuit in the state known as Canada has resulted in a state of constant urgency to stay safe and alive.

At a Canadian federal level, the authority of PHAC to dispense funding also required Indigenous collaborators. These appear to have been forged through existing administrative and professional networks. Within the institutions, and in particular the NEIHRs, personal and administrative contexts framed the commitment and support that an individual or program could provide. In a similar fashion, Indigenous governance structures such as the First Nations Indigenous Governance Centre participated in the interests of rights holding communities without being in a position of control. What can be said is that no Indigenous blood was drawn as a result of this particular attempt.

When White settlers stole Indigenous space, they also stole Indigenous time. But it is naïve to expect that somehow the urgency will decline. State and private forces disperse funds to institutions and businesses that sub-contract the labor of knowledge brokers who leverage their networks of knowledge holders and community influencers to access pieces of the Indigenous world that can be translated into data and hopefully profit. Once the data exists, the knowledge brokers – Indigenous and non-Indigenous – possess an excellent base from which to leverage national and international reputations, and their employers possess assets of multiplying returns in the era of industrial genomics. Lest we forget, Indigenous communities do not eschew non-Indigenous methods, indeed such tools may be welcome. But, increasingly, any such collaboration must be undertaken according to Indigenous-centric approaches. However, in operationalizing research, I would argue that ethnicity, in this instance Indigenous identity, is a red herring or fallacy in reasoning whereby 'Indigenous Journeys' was assumed to be inherently ethical due to the indigeneity of key personnel, notably the NPI and the IAC.[16] First, non-Indigenous individuals and groups can fully support Indigenous strategies; indeed, such is the extent and complexity of modern science-technology ecosystems that there is no other way. Second, Indigenous individuals and groups can be as guilty of incompetence, dishonesty and obfuscation.

And so, what is an Indigenous disaster research manifesto to look like? Can we assume there are robust ethical rules and regulations? Are the processes amenable to auditing and monitoring so that effective outputs and outcomes truly aid Indigenous communities in a time of urgency? Here, I will repeat principles articulated by Professor Linda Smith (1999, p. 120) who listed these 'rules' in her seminal text, *Decolonising Methodologies*, that revolve around a respect for people; personal and collective presentation and hosting yourself; generosity; cautiousness; and humility. The justification for this approach is that Indigenous Peoples assert the right to control research that purports to deal with their issues; this is the *sine quo non* of both ethical and effective research. To answer the challenge posed at the outset, what to do if you find yourself invited or instructed to research Indigenous 'issues', the default position must be to seek the ethical safety of a sovereign body. In a research context, this means engaging with sovereign Indigenous nations prior to the research proposal. Ethical and effective research (and DRR) manifestoes require accepting the rights of Indigenous Peoples to define their own needs, and how those needs are met. Ultimately, this means they take their place before the emergency arises. My call for 'time back' is a nod to Indigenous demands for 'land back' (Yellowhead Institute, 2019) and the clear need for Indigenous communities to have the time and space to understand, frame and implement their own disaster risk reduction strategies (Lambert, 2022).

The inability of PHAC, the NPI and IAC to ground 'Indigenous Journeys' in Indigenous lives is simply the denouement of colonization and its continued violence against Indigenous communities across the country that calls itself Canada. The primary risk from the incompetence of this supposedly vital – and hence urgent – proposal is the confirmation of Indigenous skepticism in future government-led pandemic responses. The rise of a 'pretendian' to the top of Canada's Indigenous academic health science likewise reveals the fraud at the heart of colonial concerns for Indigenous Peoples; the case triggered many community members's traumatic experiences of historical residential *and* contemporary graduate schools. This trauma was acknowledged in a press release announcing the indefinite leave without pay of the individual concerned in which the president of CIHR 'acknowledge[d] the pain experienced by Indigenous Peoples as a result of this matter, and would like to underscore CIHR's absolute commitment to reconciliation and continuing to *accelerate the self-determination of Indigenous Peoples in health research*' (Canadian Institutes of Health Research, 2021b, emphasis added). Given the persistence of COVID-19 infections around the world, and the lagging rates of Indigenous vaccination, establishing and then maintaining the trust and confidence of Indigenous communities is essential to the work of CIHR and other health agencies, including Indigenous health organizations. While time cannot be 'given back' to better prepare for COVID-19, calls for true Indigenous health care that would protect Indigenous communities from future fraud and pandemics can only be addressed by Indigenous sovereignty.

Conclusions

The colonial reduction of Indigenous territories has led to the majority of Indigenous communities now living in a state of actual or contrived emergency where they are at more risk from their non-Indigenous neighbors and fellow citizens from hazards and disasters. COVID-19 provides a regrettably powerful example of the embedding of vulnerabilities into Indigenous worlds. This latest pandemic revealed the conditions of vulnerability had originated with oppressive external forces, just as the authorities within health sectors remain an outcome of these histories. The flawed implementation and subsequent pulling of the 'Indigenous Journeys' seroprevalence proposal, coupled with the appointment and removal of a 'pretendian' science director, show the jurisdictions of Indigenous health in the country now called Canada remain with the non-Indigenous majority.

When colonization stole Indigenous space it also stole Indigenous time. If Indigenous vulnerability is a product of the imperial, colonial and neoliberal disaster risk creation, and if the consequent disaster landscapes are a temporal linearity, how can disaster risk reduction strategies *precede* an actual event? While each hazard presents its own specific challenges, it is clear that an Indigenous research manifesto can only break the cycle of Indigenous disasters-without-end through the acceptance of Indigenous sovereignty. As a matter of urgency, Indigenous Peoples must resume their positions of power to identify and address approaching risks to their communities in good time.

Notes

1   See Jack Goldsmith (2009) *The Terror Presidency*, Norton, p. 97.
2   Loevy builds on the work of Manin, B. (Ed.) (2008). The Emergency Paradigm and the New Terrorism. In S. Baume & B. Fontana (Eds.), *Les Usages de la Séparation des Pouvoirs* (Translation: *The Uses of the Separation of Powers*) (pp. 136–171). Michel Houdiard.
3   See https://www.thecanadianencyclopedia.ca/en/article/aboriginal-people-demography. The usual caveats on the accuracy of Indigenous statistics are particularly important in Canada where significant numbers of non-Indigenous People are claiming Indigenous heritage. See Leroux (2019) in the references.
4   Schneider v. The Queen, [1982] 2 S.C.R. 112, p. 142. Cited in Butler & Tiedemann (2011, p. 1).
5   The WHO Director-General declared the outbreak a 'public health emergency of international concern', the highest level of alarm.
6   Under the Quarantine Act, violations could be subject to a fine up to $750 000 and imprisonment of up to six months.
7   *Souverdn ist, wer ilber den Ausnahmezustand entscheidet.* Indigenous models of leadership are recognizable within ancient Roman proclamations of emergency. These conditions were normally an invasion or insurrection, or a plague or famine. A dictator was appointed who had unlimited powers, 'acting unrestrained by norm or law' (McCormick, 1997). However, as with many Indigenous approaches, there were tight constraints preventing any change or perpetual suspension of the 'regular order'.
8   McCormick presents a nuanced interpretation of Schmitt's position which, in earlier work, argued that emergency authority can only be assigned for temporary and exceptional events. McCormick (1997, p. 163) detects a shift in latter work whereby a crisis delivers a 'potentially all-powerful sovereign . . . to rescue constitutional order [and] charismatically deliver it from its own constitutional procedure'.
9   The Department of Agriculture covered federal health responsibilities from 1867 until 1919, when the Department of Health was created. https://www.canada.ca /en/health-canada/services/health-care-system/reports-publications/health-care -system/canada.html
10   https://www.canada.ca/en/intergovernmental-affairs/services/safe-restart-agreement .html
11   The Constitution Act, 1867, of Canada gave the provinces responsibility for establishing and operating hospitals, asylums and charities, while the federal government had jurisdiction over marine hospitals and quarantine. The Department of Agriculture covered federal health responsibilities from 1867 until 1919, when the Department of Health was created. https://www.canada.ca/en/health-canada /services/health-care-system/reports-publications/health-care-system/canada.html

12   I feel obliged to use the quotation marks – what some call scare quotes – to wink at a critique along the lines of 'I have reservations about using the word reservations'.
13   File 22-107.
14   The framework can be viewed here: https://www.undrr.org/publication /sendai-framework-disaster-risk-reduction-2015-2030. Witness the rebuilding of New Orleans on the same spaces with the same broad designs and methods (Blakely, 2011).
15   Recent political discourse in Canada sees the Crown's historical actions called genocidal towards First Nations, Métis and Inuit. The point was reinforced by the physical discovery of thousands of dead Indigenous children in unmarked graves across Canada.
16   At the time of writing the authenticity of a key participant as being Indigenous had been challenged.

References

Alexander, D. (2017). One Hundred Years of 'Disasterology': Looking Back and Moving Forward. *2017 CRHNet Symposium: From Catastrophe to Capacity*, Halifax, Nova Scotia.

Arriagada, P., Hahmann, T. & O'Donnell, V. (2020). *Indigenous People in Urban Areas: Vulnerabilities to the Socioeconomic Impacts of COVID-19*. Statistics Canada.

Assembly of First Nations. (2020). Annual General Assembly Final Resolutions. AFN.

Beck, U. (1992). *Risk Society: Towards a New Modernity*. Translated by M. Ritter. Sage.

Blakely, E. (2011). *The Master of Disaster*. Createspace.

Butler, M. & Tiedemann, M. (2011). The Federal Role in Health and Health Care. edited by Legal and Social Affairs Division Parliamentary Information and Research Service. Library of Parliament.

Canadian Institutes of Health Research. (2021a). NEIHR Components. https://cihr-irsc .gc.ca/e/51163.html.

Canadian Institutes of Health Research. (2021b). Statement on Institute of Indigenous Peoples' Health Scientific Director Dr. Carrie Bourassa. 1 November. https://cihr -irsc.gc.ca/e/52697.html.

COVID 19 Immunity Task Force. (2020). The COVID-19 Immunity Task Force's Mandate. COVID 19 Immunity Task Force. https://www.covid19immunitytaskforce .ca/.

COVID 19 Immunity Task Force. (2021). Dried Blood Spot Assays: A Review. CIHR. https://www.covid19immunitytaskforce.ca/dried-blood-spot-assays-a-review/.

Daschuk, J. (2013). *Clearing the Plains: Disease, Politics of Starvation, and the Loss of Aboriginal Life*. University of Regina Press.

Dunbar-Ortiz, R. (2014). *An Indigenous Peoples' History of the United States*. Beacon Press.

Eabametoong First Nation. (2019). Eabametoong First Nation Declares State of Emergency. 15 July. https://www.aptnnews.ca/wp-content/uploads/2019/07/NR -EFNSOE-July15-2019-FINAL.pdf.

Ewen, A. (Ed.) (1994). *Voice of Indigenous Peoples: Native People Address the United Nations*. Clear Light Publishers.

Franco, J. C. (2020). 'If the Virus Doesn't Kill Me . . .': Socioeconomic Impacts of COVID-19 on Rural Working People in the Global South. *Agriculture and Human Values 37*(3): 575–57. https://doi.org/10.1007/s10460-020-10073-1.

Godin, M. (2020). She Was Racially Abused by Hospital Staff as She Lay Dying. Now a Canadian Indigenous Woman's Death Is Forcing a Reckoning on Racism. *Time*. 9 October. https://time.com/5898422/joyce-echaquan-indigenous-protests-canada/.

Greenwood, M., de Leeuw, S. & Lindsay, N. (2018). Challenges in Health Equity for Indigenous Peoples in Canada. *The Lancet 391* (10131): 1645–1648.

Gregg, M. & Kneese, T. (2019). Clock as a Mediating Technology of Organization. *Media Studies 35*. https://repository.usfca.edu/ms/35.

Harris, K. (2020). Canada to Bar Entry to Travellers Who Are Not Citizens, Permanent Residents or Americans. *CBC News*. 16 March. https://www.cbc.ca/news/politics /cbsa-border-airports-screening-trudeau-covid19-coronavirus-1.5498866.

Helferty, M. et al. (2010). Incidence of Hospital Admissions and Severe Outcomes During the First and Second Waves of Pandemic (H1N1) 2009. *Canadian Medical Association Journal 182*(18): 1981–7.

Hewitt, K. (Ed.) (1983). The Idea of Calamity in a Technocratic Age. In *Interpretations of Calamity*, (pp. 3–32). Allen and Unwin.

Ingber, S. (1984). The Marketplace of Ideas: A Legitimizing Myth. *Duke Law Journal 33*(1): 1–91.

James, T. (2019). State of Emergency Declared on Makwa Sahgaiehcan First Nation After Suicides, Attempts. *Saskatoon Star Phoenix*. 23 November. https:// thestarphoenix.com/news/local-news/state-of-emergency-declared-on-makwa -sahgaiehcan-first-nation-after-suicides-attempts.

Kuiack, T. (2018). Community Resilience: Interview with Todd Kuiack. Lilia Yumagulova (Ed.). Canadian Risks and Hazards Network. http://haznet.ca /community-resilience-interview-todd-kuiack/.

Kumar, A., et al. (2009). Critically Ill Patients with 2009 Influenza A (H1N1) Infection in Canada. *Journal of the American Medical Association 302*(17): 1872–1879.

Lai, C.-C., Wang, J-H. & Hsueh. P.-R. (2020). Population-based Seroprevalence Surveys of Anti-SARS-CoV-2 Antibody: An Up-to-Date Review. *International Journal of Infectious Diseases 101*: 314–322.

Lambert, S. (2014). Māori and the Christchurch Earthquakes: The Interplay Between Indigenous Endurance and Resilience Through a Natural Disaster. *MAI Journal 3*(2): 165–180.

Lambert, S. (2022). Indigenous Communities and Disasters: A Window on Indigenous Sociology? In M. Walters, T. Kukatai, A. Gonzales and R. Henry (Eds.). *Handbook of Indigenous Sociology*. Oxford University Press (forthcoming).

Lambert, S. & Mark-Shadbolt, M. (2021). Indigenous Knowledges of Forest and Biodiversity Management: How the Watchfulness of Māori Complements and Contributes to Disaster Risk Reduction. *AlterNative: An International Journal of Indigenous Peoples 17*(2): 1–10.

Lambert, S. & Scott, J. C. (2019). International Disaster Risk Reduction Strategies and Indigenous Peoples. *International Indigenous Policy Journal 10*(2). https://doi .org/10.18584/iipj.2019.10.2.2.

Lanchester, J. (2018). Scalpers Inc. *London Review of Books 36*(11): 7–9. https://www .lrb.co.uk/v36/n11/john-lanchester/scalpers-inc.

Leo, G. (2021). Indigenous or Pretender? *CBC/Radio Canada*. 27 October. https://www .cbc.ca/newsinteractives/features/carrie-bourassa-indigenous.

Leroux, D. (2019). *Distorted Descent: White Claims to Indigenous Identity*. University of Manitoba Press.

Ling, J. (2021). Covid-19 Immunity Task Force Unable to Compile National Data. *Globe and Mail*. 27 January. https://www.theglobeandmail.com/canada /article-covid-19-immunity-task-force-unable-to-compile-national-data/.

Loevy, K. (2016). *Emergencies in Public Law: The Legal Politics of Containment*. Cambridge University Press.

Lux, M. K. (2018). *Separate Beds. 'The Government's Eyes Were Opened': The Treaty Right to Health Care*. University of Toronto Press.

McCormick, J. P. (1997). *Carl Schmitt's Critique of Liberalism: Against Politics as Technology*. Cambridge University Press.

Meadows, D. H. & Meadows, D. (2007). The History and Conclusions of the Limits to Growth. *System Dynamics Review 23* (2–3): 191–197.

Nabokov, P. (1999). *Native American Testimony: Chronicle Indian White Relations from Prophecy Present*. Penguin.

National Collaborating Centre for Aboriginal Health. (2016). *The 2009 H1N1 Influenza Pandemic Among First Nations, Inuit and Métis Peoples in Canada: Epidemiology and Gaps in Knowledge*. National Collaborating Centre for Aboriginal Health.

National Inquiry into Missing & Murdered Indigenous Women and Girls. (2019). *A Supplementary Report of the National Inquiry into Missing and Murdered Indigenous Women and Girls*. National Inquiry into Missing & Murdered Indigenous Women and Girls.

Nunn, N. (2018). Toxic Encounters, Settler Logics of Elimination, and the Future of a Continent. *Antipode 50*(5): 1330–1348.

O'Malley, V. (2012). *The Meeting Place: Māori and Pakeha Encounters, 1642–1840*. Auckland: Auckland University Press.

OHCHR/Secretariat of the Permanent Forum on Indigenous Issues. (2017). *Indigenous Peoples' Rights and the 2030 Agenda*. OHCHR; UNPFII, Division for Social Policy and Development, United Nations Department of Economic and Social Affairs. OHCHR.

Pashagumskum, J. (2021). Former AFN National Chief and Cree Grand Chief Speaks out Against Vaccine. *APTN National News*. 7 January. https://www.aptnnews .ca/national-news/former-afn-national-chief-and-cree-grand-chief-speaks-out-against -vaccine/.

Penehira, M., Green, A., Smith, L. T. & Aspin, C. (2014). Māori and Indigenous Views on R & R: Resistance and Resilience. *MAI Journal 3*(2): 96–110.

Public Health Agency of Canada. (2020). COVID-19 in Canada: Using Data and Modelling to Inform Public Health Action. Ottawa: PHAC.

Public Health Agency of Canada. (2021). *The Global Public Health Intelligence Network (GPHIN) Independent Review Panel: Final Report*. Public Health Agency, Canada (Ottawa). https://www.canada.ca/content/dam/phac-aspc/documents/corporate /mandate/about-agency/external-advisory-bodies/list/independent-review-global -public-health-intelligence-network/final-report/final-report-en.pdf.

Public Safety Canada. (2017). *An Emergency Management Framework for Canada* (3rd Ed.). Public Safety Canada.

Razack, S. (2015). *Dying from Improvement: Inquests and Inquiries into Indigenous Deaths in Custody*. University of Toronto Press.

Roache, T. & Moore, A. (2020). Fisheries Conflict: Mi'kmaw Chiefs Declare State of Emergency. *APTN News*. 18 September. https://www.aptnnews.ca/national-news /fisheries-conflict-mikmaw-chiefs-declare-state-of-emergency/.

Rolland-Harris, E., Vachon, J., Kropp, R., Frood, J., Morris, K., Pelletier, L., Rodin, R. (2012). Hospitalization of Pregnant Women with Pandemic A(H1N1) 2009 Influenza in Canada. *Epidemiology & Infection, 140*: 1316–1327.

Russell, C., Firestone, M., Kelly, L., Mushquash, C. & Fischer, B. (2016). Prescription Opioid Prescribing, Use/Misuse, Harms and Treatment Among Aboriginal People in Canada: A Narrative Review of Available Data and Indicators. *Rural and Remote Health 16*. http://www.rrh.org.au/articles/subviewnew.asp?ArticleID=3974.

Seck, P. A., Encarnacion, J. O., Tinonin, C. & Duerto-Valero, S. (2021). Gendered Impacts of COVID-19 in Asia and the Pacific: Early Evidence on Deepening Socioeconomic Inequalities in Paid and Unpaid Work. *Feminist Economics 27*(1–2): 117–132.

Shannon, T. J. (2008). *Iroquois Diplomacy on the Early American Frontier*. Penguin.

Simpson, A. (2008). Subjects of Sovereignty: Indigeneity, the Revenue Rule, and Juridics of Failed Consent. *Law and Contemporary Problems 71*(3): 191–215.

Smith, L. T. (1999). *Decolonising Methodologies: Research and Indigenous Peoples*. Zed Books.

Spielberg, S. (2012). *Lincoln*. Dreamworks Pictures.

Tait, C., Henry, B. & Walker, R. L. (2013). Child Welfare: A Social Determinant of Health for Canadian First Nations and Métis children. *Pimatisiwin: A Journal of Aboriginal and Indigenous Community Health 11*(1): 39–53.

Tait, C. L., Butt, P., Henry, R. & Bland, R. (2017). 'Our Next Generation': Moving Towards a Surveillance and Prevention Framework for Youth Suicide in Saskatchewan First Nations and Métis Populations. *Canadian Journal of Community Mental Health 36*(1): 55–65.

Tiedeman, M. (2006). Bill C-5: Public Health Agency Act of Canada. Parliamentary Information and Research Service. Library of Parliament.

Tran, D. et al. (2012). Comparison of Children Hospitalized with Seasonal Versus Pandemic Influenza. *Pediatrics 130*: 397–406.

Truth and Reconciliation Commission. (2016). *Canada's Residential Schools: The History, Part 1, Origins to 1939 – The Final Report of the Truth and Reconciliation Commission of Canada*. Vol. 1. McGill-Queen's University Press.

Turpel-Lafond, M.E. (2020). *In Plain Sight: Addressing Indigenous-specific Racism and Discrimination in B.C. Health Care*. Addressing Racism Review Summary Report, November. University of British Columbia. https://engage.gov.bc.ca/app/uploads/sites/613/2020/11/In-Plain-Sight-Full-Report.pdf.

United Nations. (2007). United Nations Declaration on the Rights of Indigenous Peoples. United Nations. https://www.un.org/development/desa/indigenouspeoples/declaration-on-the-rights-of-indigenous-peoples.html.

United Nations Conference on Trade and Development. (2020). Impact of the COVID-19 Pandemic on Trade and Development: Transitioning to a New Normal. United Nations Conference on Trade and Development (Geneva). https://unctad.org/webflyer/impact-covid-19-pandemic-trade-and-development-transitioning-new-normal.

Vera, K. B. (2012). From Papal Bull to Racial Rule: Indians of the Americas, Race, and the Foundations of International Law. *California Western International Law Journal 42*(2): 453–472.

Vogel, L. (2016). Saskatchewan Won't Declare HIV Emergency. *Canadian Medical Association Journal 188*(15): 1071–1072.

World Health Organization. (2005). Best Practices for Communicating with the Public During an Outbreak. Geneva. http://www.who.int/csr/resources/publications/WHO_CDS_2005_32web.pdf.

World Health Organization. (2021). Timeline: WHO's COVID-19 Response. Geneva. https://www.who.int/emergencies/diseases/novel-coronavirus-2019/events-as-they-happen.

Yellowhead Institute. (2019). *Land Back: A Yellowhead Institute Red Paper*. Yellowhead Institute.

6   A post-COVID-19 research agenda for disaster prevention, response and research

Cordula Dittmer and Daniel F. Lorenz

Introduction

While there is much talk of an imminent end to the COVID-19 pandemic, we argue in the following that, instead of a final end, we rather expect a 'Pandemocene' in which social, political or economic processes are continuously interpreted in light of the COVID-19 pandemic. Accordingly, the COVID-19 pandemic will also influence disaster research, prevention and response. To understand these implications in more detail, we first define the ways in which the pandemic can be understood as a disaster and present the complexity of future disasters given fundamental shifts in the interaction of social processes. Following this, we focus on practical, ethical, thematic and conceptual implications for research and, in the context of prevention and response, on implications for the operational level, the individual and organizational resilience of disaster relief organizations and the level of aid recipients.

What is the 'post' in post-COVID-19?

Since the onset of the COVID-19 pandemic—reinforced especially by the first lockdown in spring 2020—some scientific and sociopolitical actors (in the Global North) have expressed hope for, or expectations of, a profound change in society post–COVID-19 (see the chapters by Matthewman and Goode on this). These hopes relate, for instance, to an increase in attention to climate change and its disastrous impacts on societies and their economic systems (Milner et al., 2021) or to the possibility of new social and political orders (Lorenz & Dittmer, 2020; Leach et al., 2021). After a year of comprehensive and profound changes in the social realm, isolation through contact restrictions, the effects of infections, massive travel restrictions and the shift of network activities to the virtual sphere, fundamental questions about the consequences for a post–COVID-19 world also arise for science. These are flanked by currents from the Black Lives Matter movement and the de- and/or postcolonial critique accompanying it, which question the power relations of researchers but also dominant theories and concepts within the academic community (for disaster research see, for example, Meding et al., 2020).

In the early 1990s, in the context of socioecological and transdisciplinary research, science-and-technology studies, or discussions in the context of the Anthropocene, ideas were already being developed about what science in a 'post-normal age' (Funtowicz & Ravetz, 1993) could look like:

> The reductionist, analytical worldview which divides systems into ever smaller elements, studied by ever more esoteric specialism, is being replaced by a systemic, synthetic and humanistic approach. The old dichotomies of facts and values, and of knowledge and ignorance, are being transcended. Natural systems are recognized as dynamic and complex; those involving interactions with humanity are 'emergent', including properties of reflection and contradiction. The science appropriate to this new condition will be based on the assumptions of unpredictability, incomplete control, and a plurality of legitimate perspectives. (Funtowicz & Ravetz, 1993, p. 739)

What do all these academic developments mean for disaster research, disaster management and preparedness in a post–COVID-19 society, in which, as in no other time since World War II, the pandemic has exposed fractures, fragilities and vulnerabilities and made them visible worldwide through global interconnectedness?

Here, it seems helpful to first ask what could constitute a post–COVID-19 society at all. After these profound worldwide changes and experiences, how realistic is it to be able to speak of a post–COVID-19 society in the near future (see also Goode in this collection)? Would it be more sensible to assume that the experiences of the last months—and those that will follow—have inscribed themselves into the majority of societal and social bodies and into politics, economics, art and so on, to such an extent that, strictly speaking, there will be no 'after' at all and that societal experiences will still be framed by the pandemic and the pandemic experiences for a long time (Wynn and Trnka's chapter also discusses issues of futurity and temporality)? Homi K. Bhabha (1994, pp. 1–2) writes in his seminal book on postcolonial currents, *The Location of Culture*:

> Our existence today is marked by a tenebrous sense of survival, living on the borderlines of the 'present', for which there seems to be no proper name other than the

current and controversial shiftiness of the prefix 'post' [. . .] we find ourselves in the moment of transit where space and time cross to produce complex figures of difference and identity, past and present, inside and outside, inclusion and exclusion.

Of course, in these descriptions, Bhabha refers to the discussions of postmodernism, poststructuralism and postcolonialism that have been emerging since the 1980s, critiques of homogenizing and exclusionary categories whose historical continuities are far more extensive and profound than the current phase of the pandemic. Nevertheless, in addressing the question of how to think about disasters in the face of a pandemic, it seems useful to include this idea here: We are precisely not in a synchronous sequence of different ages (or steps in the pandemic response), instead, we observe a complex interplay of different temporalities, vulnerabilities, escalation dynamics and discontinuities that cannot be declared to have ended at any particular point in time. Who is affected, how and why, how the crisis is managed, which measures affect whom and how intensely and who is the winner or loser in each phase can hardly be determined uniformly in the COVID-19 pandemic.

Some virologists (for example, Morens & Fauci, 2020) are already proclaiming that the world has entered a pandemic era, as global environmental degradation and climate change have radically increased the likelihood of zoonotic disease transmission, that is, the transmission of viruses from animals to humans, and thus also the likelihood of pandemics even more devastating than the COVID-19 pandemic (see Wallace and Wallace in this collection). From a virological point of view, therefore, it cannot be assumed that the pathogen will disappear. The genetic successors of the last major pandemic, the so-called Spanish Flu of 1918, are responsible for a large number of deaths worldwide to this day. However, this has rarely been discussed academically or publicly. Although there are accounts of the historical significance of pandemics in the Middle Ages (cf. McNeill, 1976), the effects of past pandemics such as the so-called Spanish Flu on the social processes of the last century have hardly been researched and socially discussed to date. Only Laura Spinney (2017) has demonstrated clearly how complexly the Spanish Flu of 1918 challenged social and political systems worldwide and how its social consequences continue to shape the present.

The COVID-19 pandemic, we argue, will not simply end at a defined point in time; rather, we see the necessity for future scientific discussions that assume a Pandemocene in which social, political or economic processes are seen, experienced and interpreted in light of the COVID-19 pandemic—not only on a rational level but as habitually inscribed in the different bodies of society. Accordingly, we see the need to address the ongoing impact and reinterpretation of 2020, 2021 and beyond in the context of multiple developments, including future pandemics and (other) disasters.

The COVID-19 pandemic as a disaster?

Before answering the question of what disaster research and response might look like in the Pandemocene, it is important to clarify whether a pandemic is, strictly speaking, the subject of disaster research at all and whether the field should not rather be left to other scientific communities, for example, crisis researchers (Boin et al., 2018). To put it differently, which aspects or approaches qualify disaster research as the appropriate context in which to analyze the pandemic? This question arises at this point because many definitions of disaster still refer to the core characteristics of Charles Fritz's (1961, p. 655) classical definition that conceptualizes a disaster as a rapid onset 'event, concentrated in time and space,' although the concept has been the subject of many debates (Perry & Quarantelli, 2005; Quarantelli, 2006). The pandemic, however, eludes such a standardized concept of disaster, as we will show in the following.

Historically, pandemics are not a new phenomenon and are therefore present in disaster research and in disaster response and preparedness. However, as in many other fields, there are various interpretations and approaches regarding how pandemics are classified and analyzed in the categories of established social science disaster research and thus in research on complex disasters in the Pandemocene.

In the transatlantic sociology of disasters, Quarantelli et al. (2007) dealt with the question of how pandemics can be conceptualized in disaster sociology, especially against the background of new types of (complex) crises and disasters, in the face of the first Severe Acute Respiratory Syndrome (SARS) epidemic in 2003. The authors define six characteristics that distinguish this epidemic as a new type of disaster and crisis, which they call 'trans-system social rupture': (1) Crossing of nation state, functional, sectoral and so on, boundaries; (2) extremely rapid spread and simultaneous global awareness of the risk due to high media presence, the end being difficult to foresee or define; (3) the cause is difficult to trace and the course and effects are difficult to predict, resulting in high ambiguity; (4) potential numbers of direct and indirect victims are highly difficult to determine; (5) coping on the local level and often even at the national level is not possible, and only international and transnational organizations can cope with this challenge; and (6) the presence of large numbers of emergent actions and actors, especially related to informal social networks or virtual communities, that are difficult to recognize from the outside. Fundamental to these arguments (and to the debates in US disaster sociology) is the approach taken by Quarantelli (2000)—and later further elaborated on by Fischer (2003)—who introduced the distinction between emergencies, disasters and catastrophes[1] as damaging events of different qualities. Also fundamental are his basic assumptions that disasters are social processes represented via social disruption and damage (for an overview, see Perry, 2007). Quarantelli (2005, p.335) argued, however, with regard to the AIDS epidemic, against classifying epidemics per se as disasters: 'Personally, we are inclined to exclude from the concept of "disaster" all very diffused events, including traditional droughts and famines and certain kinds of epidemics . . . it is best to think of the concept of a disaster as an occasion involving an immediate crisis or emergency.' This view was criticized by, among others, Hsu (2019), who emphasizes that the temporality and crisis-like nature of disruptive phenomena are perceived very differently in different social contexts.

In a first attempt to capture the current COVID-19 pandemic within the established sociological categories of disaster research, Montano and Savitt (2020) concluded: 'The existing categories of emergencies, disasters, and catastrophes, as they are currently conceptualized, exclude certain events. Epidemics and pandemics, because their characteristics differ so significantly from the traditional understanding of natural and technological hazard types, break the bounds of the classification structure, and challenge the traditional thinking.' Yamori and Goltz (2021) also agree that the pandemic is a '"nondisaster" according to prevailing concepts.' Kelman (2020) argues in the opposite direction and considers the pandemic (yet another) proof that there are no natural disasters and that disasters are therefore social phenomena through and through—and thus, by extension, the subject of disaster research.

In his article 'Offene Fragen der Seuchensoziologie' ('Open Questions in the Sociology of Epidemics'), Lars Clausen (1985)—one of the first disaster sociologists in the German-speaking world—was concerned with the question of whether pandemics represent the disaster par excellence, if disasters are defined as social processes 'which proceed very rapidly,[2] very radically affect all social spheres, and trigger non-scientific causal explanations' (Clausen 1985, p.247, own translation). From a sociological point of view, Clausen defines five descriptive aspects that, in his opinion, characterize 'new epidemics.' First, a completely new quality of damage occurs: Previous epidemics have become so integrated either into everyday life or into normal social processes (domesticated) that normalizing rituals, and later also vaccinations, were developed, which made dealing with them a part of everyday life. Second, suffering and unexpected death are banished in secularized societies. Institutionalized forms of coping hardly exist anymore, and epidemics are no longer taken for granted. Rather, they 'irrupt' without having causally derivable explanations, such as the belief of earlier times that 'illness is God's punishment.' Third, the acceleration of societal developments such as exponential population growth and interconnectedness (industrialization, migration, mass tourism and so on) have massively increased exposure to infectious diseases. Fourth, possible modes of infection have become more diverse through the production of biological warfare agents in laboratories and the storage of pathogens of diseases such as the plague and through emerging antibiotic resistance. Fifth, new infection routes develop in modern societies that, for instance, could be exploited by terrorist groups.

Clausen argues for abandoning the analytic division of 'everyday life—event—everyday life' and instead asks how extreme events are socially embedded in everyday life and result from the very processes of everyday life. For a sociology of epidemics, he focuses on the questions of how modern societies can deal with human failures such as suffering and death when there is no longer any meaningful 'divine' explanation for them and how social figurations (Norbert Elias' word for mutual dependencies) structure epidemic threats or, in other words, whether preventive disaster control measures develop counterinduced effects when they are effective in one place but produce secondary effects in other places that were not initially considered.

Although Clausen's remarks originated 40 years ago entirely in the shadow of the Cold War, they seem surprisingly up to date for the analysis of the current pandemic. His fundamental call to understand the conditions of the emergence and eradication of epidemics as a constitutive part of everyday life rather than as extreme events is also reflected in the proposal to conceive of future disaster research within a Pandemocene (for more on the future of disaster research see Lambert's contribution to this publication). Clausen goes much further here and also sees the history and development of social processes in retrospect as variously conditioned by epidemics and their management.

In summary, conceptual sociological approaches already conceived in the 1980s can also be applied to the analysis of the current pandemic and allow the COVID-19 pandemic to be clearly defined as a disaster in this sense: The COVID-19 pandemic is a transnational phenomenon that can only be managed transnationally. Although there is already extensive historical knowledge of epidemics and pandemics in individual Western societies (for example, analysis of the Spanish Flu), this knowledge is not well acknowledged on a large scale because vaccinations have banished the handling of these events, as well as the associated suffering and mass death, from societal consciousness. In principle, communicable diseases, like other threats to the social order, have become (supposedly) controllable. The pandemic crosses functionally differentiated boundaries—all individuals and social systems (health, economic, educational, cultural and so on) are affected (as reflected in the Greek *pan*, meaning 'all,' and *demos*, meaning 'the people') and spread worldwide at breakneck speed. However, because of these broad impacts, a variety of (emergent) actors are necessary and actually deployed in response, who did not play major roles in disaster management hitherto (entire nation-state governments, health systems, financial systems, research and so on). Knowledge about the course and effects of pandemics exists not only at the conceptual level but also at the level of disaster management, where a large number of concepts originated during the Cold War and were updated after 9/11, although they primarily dealt with the effects of biological attacks. These insights into the capabilities and performance of disaster management differ little from those needed for current management of the COVID-19 pandemic. With respect to the issue of temporality that Quarantelli and others see as a central feature of why pandemics tend not to be disasters in the conventional sense, we argue that the pandemic is a disastrous process that includes in its temporal course both rapid-onset moments and slowly evolving phases.

Thus, the pandemic is not a black swan, and while its management is exhausting and protracted and there is a lack of resources and/or capabilities in many places, it is not so complex that there is a lack of knowledge about consequences and ways of coping. Nevertheless, the pandemic highlights the characteristics of the disasters to come. It therefore seems appropriate to ask what future disasters in the Pandemocene will look like and how they can be countered, both in terms of research and in terms of preparedness and response.

Complex disasters as the new normal

In the COVID-19 pandemic, it has become abundantly clear that there is a lack of societal coping skills; moreover, the impact of the infection dynamics in all areas of society is extreme and, in turn, increasingly complex. Decisive for this increase in complexity are the side effects, interactions and consequences of societal processes at different levels. Researchers speak, for example, of reflexive modernity (Beck et al., 2003), (world) risk society (Beck, 2009) and, recently, the Anthropocene (Dominey-Howes, 2018). The increase in social complexity corresponds to an increase in the complexity of the catastrophes that have been diagnosed (de Smet et al., 2012). Disasters cannot be understood as causes but only as (social) effects (Dombrowsky, 1995), since 'disasters . . . are characteristic rather than accidental features of the places and societies where they occur' (Hewitt, 1983, p. 25). Thus, disasters do not necessarily become more complex and global because hazards change or trigger each other (cf. McGuire, 2012) but mainly because the complexity of the causal systems, meaning societies, has changed radically in the last decades.

Manifestations of '"modern disasters" or "disasters of the 21st century"' (de Smet et al., 2012, p. 138) can be observed more often. In the Fukushima triple disaster,[3] for instance, various social processes, such as the interaction of natural hazards, high-risk technologies, demographic change and inadequate protection and coping capabilities, were particularly catastrophic (Ranghieri & Ishiwatari, 2014). Modern disasters show different and specific dynamics of social change when, on the one hand, the dangers threatening security are multiplied by manifold and partially decoupled processes of change and, on the other hand, the social coping capacities (institutionalized in disaster control) do not change adequately (Dombrowsky, 1995; Oliver-Smith, 1999).

In the *New Dark Age*, James Bridle (2019, p. 46) also describes an epistemological paradox that has relevance for disasters, especially modern ones. 'The more obsessively we attempt to compute the world, the more unknowably complex it appears.' He explains how increasing, ever more differentiated bodies of knowledge and new technologies generate vast amounts of data and use them for increasingly autonomous control processes that are increasingly perceived as superior to human planning (cf. automation bias). This results in new epistemic blind spots and, thus, incomprehensible systemic interactions that can have catastrophic effects, both individually and collectively. According to Bridle (2019, p. 14), 'like climate change, the effects of technology are widespread across the globe and are already affecting every area of our lives. These effects are potentially catastrophic and result from an inability to comprehend the turbulent and networked outputs of our own inventions.' Given the existing trajectories, we can expect further exacerbation of the problem in the years ahead: 'As more complex solutions are brought to bear on ever more complex problems, we risk even greater systemic problems being overlooked' (Bridle, 2019, p. 101). Bridle—in line with Hewitt's (1983) critique—points out how a technocratic disaster paradigm not only obscures our view of disasters but can produce them on a previously unknown scale.

To date, the focus of disaster prevention and disaster management has predominantly been on high-frequency natural (heavy precipitation, storms, floods and so on) and technological (explosions, chemical spills and so on) hazards, but less tangible, slow-building threats to security such as droughts or rare events such as pandemics are increasingly being considered. However, the praxis here seems to be several years behind the scientific debate, as disaster research has turned much more consciously to slow disasters or gradual-onset disasters (Hsu, 2019; Knowles, 2014; Staupe-Delgado, 2019) and rare events. Although there is much talk of an all-hazards approach in disaster management, which can also be applied to pandemics (cf. Penta et al., 2021), in practice, this approach usually deals with separately considered hazards (Komendantova et al., 2014) or levels out differences in the ways they are dealt with (Lorenz & Voss, 2013). Such approaches—one could also speak of the dominant view with Hewitt (1983)—thus disregard complex interaction effects as well as social dynamics, the integration of which is necessary for the successful management of disasters in the twenty-first century. Relief in the context of disasters is still limited to basic needs and the return to a predisaster state; this is also an expression of a still-present event-based understanding of disasters that has been criticized for quite some time (cf. Matthewman, 2015). Even less attention is given to systemic hazards that arise genuinely through social processes or that superimpose and amplify other risks and hazards (Kasperson et al., 1988).

Implications for future disaster research and response

All of this has multiple implications for future disaster research and management. 'The future is not the past repeated' wrote Quarantelli (1996) with regard to future disasters. It is therefore true that 'disaster research must change with the times' (Matthewman, 2015, p. 6). On the one hand, the subject matter is changing radically; on the other hand, novel approaches to the practice of disaster management are needed. The following remarks, however, are to be understood only as a necessarily incomplete list, since future disasters will always be an 'empirical falsification' (Dombrowsky, 1995, p. 241) of our current disaster planning.

Disaster research

With regard to disaster research, we differentiate practical and ethical implications for research, on the one hand, and thematic and conceptual implications, on the other. These implications underline former research agendas for disaster research (Quarantelli, 1996, 2005; Tierney, 2007, 2019) to some extent, but also go beyond them in some respects.

Practical and ethical implications for research

In terms of research practice and ethics, the question arises as to how empirical research in a Pandemocene can take place at all or whether it should, given the researchers' own involvement in the pandemic (see the chapters in this collection by Wynn and Trnka; and Southerton, Clark, Watson and Lupton). The lack of access, or at least limited access, to the field affects the previously used research methodology (Stallings, 2002) in many ways and thus also the results and their comparability with previous findings. In terms of research practice, in the short term, the uneven distribution of affectedness and the availability of vaccines means that there are fewer opportunities for field research, particularly in non-Western societies. In the middle term, social disparities in research might be exacerbated. While researchers in the Global North are expected to be vaccinated in the near future and can rely on health protection systems in the background, others, especially researchers in the Global South, will still be at massive risk or affected by local containment measures. While (social science) disaster researchers face these problems even in the absence of a pandemic, they are vastly exacerbated in the pandemic context. Additionally, 'research fatigue' has already been diagnosed (Patel et al., 2020) in the context of research on COVID-19, which could make data collection difficult.

Thematic and conceptual implications

Social science research on disasters began approximately 100 years ago with the study of the Halifax explosion by Samuel H. Prince (1920) and found a new focus at the end of World War II and during the Cold War, transforming again at the turn of the millennium (Tierney, 2007). Despite these changes, the core of the research was based on a paradigm that conceptualized threats and impacts in a comparatively linear fashion based on known hazards and consequences. The fundamental shifts that have occurred therefore call for a critical reevaluation of empirical knowledge in disaster research. The question arises as to whether the foundations and findings of disaster research that were valid for the past decades can still claim validity in the Pandemocene: Which findings have generally outlived their usefulness, and what will be different in the future? Thus, the often criticized (Tierney, 2019) but still dominant (Hsu, 2019) event centeredness in the conceptualization of disasters (cf., for example, Fritz's [1961] classic definition of disaster as cited earlier) is completely unsuitable for understanding disasters as multiform, temporally and spatially decoupled destruction processes. This has implications not only for the definition of disasters but also for related theorems and well-known and widespread middle-range theories, such as 'emergent groups' (Stallings & Quarantelli,

1985) or 'convergence' (Heide, 2003), which seem to be based on a temporally sequenced and spatially delimited understanding of disasters and need to be critically reexamined in the context of the pandemic as well as with regard to complex disasters (Lorenz & Dittmer, 2020).

Scientific discourse has long recognized different degrees of severity and temporalities of disasters (Fischer, 2003; Quarantelli, 2000) and is increasingly beginning to integrate complex interaction effects as well (de Smet et al., 2012). Thus, there is talk of 'compound disasters' (Wachira, 1997), which refers to when 'different, but related, disaster-agents' interact in disasters (cf. also Funabashi & Kitazawa, 2012). So-called natech disasters (natural hazard triggering technological disasters) and techna disasters (technology trigging natural hazards, Gill & Ritchie, 2018) represent the interaction effects of natural and technological hazards that cause increasingly complex disasters. Pescaroli and Alexander (2015, p. 65) refer to the Tōhoku earthquake of 11 March 2011 as a 'cascading disaster.' Such disasters are defined as

> extreme events, in which cascading effects increase in progression over time and generate unexpected secondary events of strong impact. These tend to be at least as serious as the original event, and to contribute significantly to the overall duration of the disaster's effects. [. . .] Cascading disasters tend to highlight unresolved vulnerabilities in human society. In cascading disasters one or more secondary events can be identified and distinguished from the original source of disaster.

More recently, 'consecutive disasters' (de Ruiter et al., 2020, p. 2) have gained attention; these denote 'two or more disasters that occur in succession, and whose direct impacts overlap spatially before recovery from a previous event is considered to be completed.'

In this sense, disasters are to be understood as long-term, interacting phenomena that are not easily reduced to individual factors. Thus, for instance, 'natural hazards' will be only one factor among many contributors to catastrophes and will thereby continue to lose their naturalness and increasingly emerge as a socially produced variable (cf. the debates about the Anthropocene [Dominey-Howes, 2018] or the importance of climate change or resource extraction for geophysical processes [McGuire, 2012; Tierney, 2019]). Rather, disasters will increasingly emerge as escalating disruptive effects and mutually reinforcing damage in all areas of society, whereby future catastrophic damage may increasingly manifest itself beyond primary effects such as direct deaths, injuries and those directly affected (Quarantelli, 1996). Accordingly, social science more broadly, as well as interdisciplinary expertise, will be needed to understand disasters (cf. Tierney, 2007).

Furthermore, the spectrum of disastrous temporalities is broadening: In addition to rapid-onset disasters, we can expect an increase in slow destructive processes in the form of slow disasters (Knowles, 2014). These fast and slow disasters will increasingly interact and overlap in the future. Fortun (2013, as cited in Knowles, 2014, p. 778) speaks in this context of 'increasing incidence of both acute disaster—such as BP's Deepwater Horizon disaster, the Fukushima disaster, or the Bhopal disaster—and chronic, slow disaster, which almost always follows acute disaster, but also can emerge separately, and more quietly.' The same applies to different levels of disaster severity: The distinction between emergencies, disasters and catastrophes (Quarantelli, 2000) could increasingly fade as interdependencies increase, for instance, in the context of consecutive events.

All in all, these radical changes in the subject matter require both altered epistemic foundations and new instruments of empirical research. Thus, the question 'What is a disaster?' negotiated in several anthologies and essays at the end of the last century (Quarantelli 2006; Perry & Quarantelli, 2005) arises again with renewed poignancy in the face increasing loss of socially accepted conceptions of normality or increasingly socially disparate expectations regarding normal social change. Ultimately, this will also require the incorporation of entirely new strands of research within disaster studies or the development of new disaster sociological theory, although these are difficult to envisage today.

Prevention and response

All this has decisive consequences for dealing with disasters and catastrophic risks. Thus, disaster management, as the handling of damage that has occurred, and risk management, as the minimization of future damage, are increasingly amalgamating. This also has profound implications for established concepts for dealing with disasters in planning. The disaster management cycle, for instance, while not without criticism for its phases—preparedness, response, recovery and mitigation—is still a central heuristic tool of disaster management. As the contours of catastrophic events continue to unravel, so do the phases: Preparedness, response, recovery and mitigation not only overlap but also become fully blurred in complex disasters. Yamori and Goltz (2021, p. 12) refer to the COVID-19 pandemic as "response-recovery cycles' in which measures assumed to reduce infections are implemented, appear to be working, and recovery is being achieved only to witness renewed surges in infections, prompting a return to response measures.' What preparation for future situations is, what coping with current problems is and what reconstruction and aftercare are simply become indistinguishable in the face of complex disasters.

Despite the dissolution of boundaries, implications for different aspects of prevention and response can nevertheless be characterized. Complex disasters, such as the COVID-19 pandemic, mean that prevention must be thought of much more broadly. When complex disasters affect all sectors of society due to extensive interconnectedness and sometimes unpredictable interactions, disaster risk reduction thus becomes a cross-cutting task for all sectors of society.

Response

Implications can also be identified in the context of disaster management. In the following, we will focus on three different areas: the operational and tactical level, the individual and organizational resilience of disaster relief organizations and the level of aid recipients.

At the operational-tactical level, one expectation is that in the future, disaster response will no longer be local and temporally limited but will cross known temporal and spatial boundaries (Yamori & Goltz, 2021; de Smet et al., 2012). This makes practices of 'zoning' as well as associated notions of materiality and causality that have worked well in disaster management in the past more or less useless (Matthewman, 2015).

The temporally and spatially ramified effects and the associated unclear attribution of the damage (see also below) also complicate the political and strategic management of these events (de Smet et al., 2012). 'Slow-onset disasters like the coronavirus pandemic . . . present challenges in explaining these complex hazards in that experts may not be readily identifiable, key elements in understanding the hazards may be unknown and clear pathways to effective response may be unavailable' (Yamori & Goltz, 2021, p. 14). Thus, protective measures are much more difficult to communicate and may be instrumentalized accordingly in a politicizing manner in the context of 'invisible' complex hazards and unknown cascading effects.

Moreover, as complex disasters increasingly transcend boundaries of time and space as well as boundaries of societal differentiation (Tierney, 2019), an increasing number of actors are needed to (successfully) cope with them. However, the necessary collaboration is also becoming more complex, as the massive impact of disasters on all sectors of society increasingly requires collaboration with actors who are not otherwise involved with crises and disasters on a day-to-day basis. For example, cooperation between health and disaster management actors during the COVID-19 pandemic has been challenging, as was that between asylum and migration authorities on the one hand and civil protection and humanitarian aid actors on the other during the 2015/16 European refugee crisis (Dittmer & Lorenz, 2019). The expected greater geographic extent alone increasingly implies the need for not only interorganizational but also cross-border cooperation. In the future, even more complex constellations of actors can be expected (Bragg, 2015). Accordingly, broad societal preparation of all functional areas for disasters and the necessary interorganizational cooperation will have to take place.

However, it is not only the actors that change in complex disasters but also the demands on them. Complex disasters point to the increasing need for anticipatory procedures as well as the consideration of complex interactions, which have thus far hardly been the focus of what is essentially technical-material damage control and disaster management. Although initial efforts are beginning to emerge at the international level (Weingärtner & Wilkinson, 2019), a fundamental paradigm shift is still a long way off, and the question also arises as to which new blind spots are associated with such approaches (cf. the comments on automation bias above).

While many industrialized nations have become accustomed to disaster management that functions well in many areas—with all the improvements that are always possible—there is a threat of previously unknown resource and personnel bottlenecks in the face of complex hazards and escalating disasters. This also raises the question of how operational tactics as well as decision-making processes will evolve under the constraints of scarce resources and how to deal in the future with the corresponding problem situations, some of which have already arisen in the pandemic, such as necessary prioritization or triage situations.

It must also be assumed that organizations and emergency personnel will be much more affected by disasters themselves. The COVID-19 pandemic shows, for example, the limits of disaster relief organizations' ability to act if they themselves do not have sufficient personal protective equipment or if members are themselves in quarantine or even fall ill. Accordingly, the individual and organizational resilience of disaster relief organizations will have to be given much greater consideration in planning processes in the future.

If novel types of disaster, especially those caused by human beings, represent a 'new species of trouble' (Erikson, 1995) it must also be expected that the changes outlined will have far-reaching consequences for those affected and those receiving assistance. A key 'feature of the disasters of the 21st century is that they have a more devastating impact on society, with more infrastructures destroyed and more people affected' (de Smet et al., 2012, pp. 139–40). On the one hand, research has become increasingly better at analyzing the ramified effects of disasters in the form of primary, secondary and tertiary impacts, and research can clearly trace the 'ratchet effect' (Chambers, 1983) of disasters. On the other hand, in view of the expected disasters, a completely new form of fuzziness is looming if, for instance, rapid- and gradual-onset disasters on different spatial scales interact. This has the consequence that, increasingly, effects of a secondary or tertiary nature are difficult to determine (cf. Nixon, 2011), and in general, the boundaries between primary, secondary and tertiary impacts are increasingly lost (cf. Yamori & Goltz, 2021) and entirely new, hitherto unknown, vulnerabilities are becoming apparent. As a consequence, it must be expected that rescue, relief and reconstruction programs will be increasingly less able to identify the most vulnerable and other potential beneficiaries, and new, currently unknown vulnerabilities will emerge. In addition, the focus of such programs must be adapted if it can no longer be assumed that any kind of return to the status quo ante disaster is possible. Rather, these programs will need to focus not solely on reconstruction but also on the upcoming consecutive events (de Ruiter et al., 2020) and the required preparedness.

Conclusion

As our discussion has shown, the implications of a post–COVID-19 society for disaster research, preparedness and response are extremely complex. We have argued that the experience of the COVID-19 pandemic is unlikely to disappear from societal memory in the near future, and therefore, we anticipate that we will face a new age, the Pandemocene. Against this backdrop, however, it is not the pandemic per se that challenges disaster research, management and preparedness but rather an increase in complex disasters in general. These have been diagnosed by researchers for some years, but the findings and challenges have not yet reached disaster management and preparedness. Here, an outdated event-centered concept of disaster continues to be used to the greatest possible extent. Thus, there are a multitude of challenges at different levels, the effects of which are still difficult to foresee.

Notes

1   In this distinction emergencies are everyday events such as accidents that require the planned response of rescue personnel. Disasters differ from emergencies in at least four ways: A disaster involves mass convergence, that is, the convergence of a

large number of organizations on the scene. In a disaster these organizations need to adjust to losing autonomy, different performance standards and operate a closer interface with the public and private sectors. Catastrophes—compared with a disaster—involve heavily impacted community infrastructures, the interruption of community functions, the inability of local officials to fulfill their usual work and that nearby communities are themselves unable to provide any help. Additionally, media coverage is much higher and the political arena becomes much more involved (Quarantelli, 2000).

2   Whereby the time dimension must not be seen in absolute terms but in relation to societal perceptions and collective coping capacities.

3   The disaster involved three interacting hazards. The most powerful earthquake ever recorded in Japan triggered powerful tsunami waves that contributed to the meltdown in the Fukushima Daiichi powerplant. While the region was well prepared for earthquakes, it was not so well prepared for the subsequent tsunami waves and the meltdown in the Fukushima Daiichi powerplant.

References

Beck, U. (2009). *Risk Society: Towards a New Modernity*. Sage.

Beck, U., Bonss, W., & Lau, C. (2003). 'The Theory of Reflexive Modernization.' *Theory, Culture & Society 20* (2), 1–33.

Bhabha, H. K. (1994). *The Location of Culture*. Routledge.

Boin, A., 't Hart, P., & Kuipers, S. (2018). 'The Crisis Approach.' In H. Rodríguez, W. Donner, & J. Trainor (Eds.) *Handbook of Disaster Research* (Second Edition) (pp. 23–38). Springer.

Bragg, C. (2015). 'Disaster Management and Multilateral Humanitarian Aid: Parallelism Vs. Combined Forces.' In P. Gibbons, & H.-J. Heintze (Eds.) *The Humanitarian Challenge: 20 Years European Network on Humanitarian Action (NOHA)* (pp. 1–16). Springer.

Bridle, J. (2019). *New Dark Age: Technology and the End of the Future*. Verso.

Chambers, R. (1983). *Rural Development: Putting the Last First*. Longman.

Clausen, L. (1985). 'Offene Fragen der Seuchensoziologie.' ['Open Questions in the Sociology of Epidemics.'] *Österreichische Zeitschrift für Soziologie 10* (3+4), 241–9.

Dittmer, C., & Lorenz, D. F. (2019). 'Disaster Situation and Humanitarian Emergency – In-Between Responses to the Refugee Crisis in Germany.' *International Migration*. https://doi.org/10.1111/imig.12679.

Dombrowsky, W. R. (1995). 'Again and Again: Is a 'Disaster' What We Call Disaster? Some Conceptual Notes on Conceptualizing the Object of Disaster Sociology.' *International Journal of Mass Emergencies and Disasters 13* (3), 241–54.

Dominey-Howes, D. (2018). 'Hazards and Disasters in the Anthropocene: Some Critical Reflections for the Future.' *Geoscience Letters 5* (1), 611.

Erikson, K. (1995). *A New Species of Trouble. The Human Experience of Modern Disasters*. Norton.

Fischer, H. W. (2003). 'The Sociology of Disaster: Definitions, Research Questions, & Measurements' Continuation of the Discussion in a Post-September 11 Environment.' *International Journal of Mass Emergencies and Disasters 21* (1), 91–107.

Fritz, C. E. (1961). 'Disaster.' In R. K. Merton & R.A Nisbet (Eds.) *Contemporary Social Problems* (pp. 651–94). Harcourt, Brace & World.

Funabashi, Y., & Kitazawa, K. (2012). 'Fukushima in Review: A Complex Disaster, a Disastrous Response.' *Bulletin of the Atomic Scientists 68* (2), 9–21.

Funtowicz, S. O., & Ravetz, J. O. (1993). 'Science for the Post-Normal Age.' *Futures 25* (7), 739–55.

Gill, D. A., & Ritchie, L. A. (2018). 'Contributions of Technological and Natech Disaster Research to the Social Science Disaster Paradigm.' In H. Rodríguez, W. Donner, & J. Trainor (Eds.) *Handbook of Disaster Research* (Second Edition) (pp. 39–60). Springer.

Heide, E. (2003). 'Convergence Behavior in Disasters.' *Annals of Emergency Medicine 41* (4), 463–66.

Hewitt, K. (1983). 'The Idea of Calamity in a Technocratic Age.' In K. Hewitt (Ed.) *Interpretations of Calamity: From the Viewpoint of Human Ecology* (pp. 2–32). Allen & Unwin.

Hsu, E. L. (2019). 'Must Disasters Be Rapidly Occurring? The Case for an Expanded Temporal Typology of Disasters.' *Time & Society 28* (3), 904–21.

Kasperson, R. E., Renn, O., Slovic, P., Brown, H. S., Emel, J., Goble, R., Kasperson, J. X., & Ratick, S. (1988). 'The Social Amplification of Risk: A Conceptual Framework.' *Risk Analysis 8* (2), 177–87.

Kelman, I. (2020). 'COVID-19: What Is the Disaster?' *Social Anthropology 28* (2), 296–7.

Knowles, S. G. (2014). 'Learning from Disaster? The History of Technology and the Future of Disaster Research.' *Technology and Culture 55* (4), 773–84.

Komendantova, N., Mrzyglocki, R., Mignan, A., Khazai, B., Wenzel, F., Patt, A., & Fleming, K. (2014). 'Multi-Hazard and Multi-Risk Decision-Support Tools as a Part of Participatory Risk Governance: Feedback from Civil Protection Stakeholders.' *International Journal of Disaster Risk Reduction 8*, 50–67.

Leach, M., MacGregor, H., Scoones, I., & Wilkinson, A. (2021). 'Post-Pandemic Transformations: How and Why COVID-19 Requires Us to Rethink Development.' *World Development 138*: 105233.

Lorenz, D. F., & Dittmer, C. (2020). '(Disaster) Utopian Moments in the Pandemic: A European Perspective.' *Items: Insights from the Social Sciences.* Social Science Research Council. https://items.ssrc.org/covid-19-and-the-social-sciences/disaster-studies /disaster-utopian-moments-in-the-pandemic-a-european-perspective/.

Lorenz, D. F., & Voss, M. (2013). '"Not a Political Problem": Die Bevölkerung Im Diskurs Um Kritische Infrastrukturen.' ['Not a Political Problem': The Population in the Discourse on Critical Infrastructure]. In L. Hempel, M. Bartels, & T. Markwart (Eds.) *Aufbruch Ins Unversicherbare: Zum Katastrophendiskurs Der Gegenwart* [Departure into the Uninsurable: On the Contemporary Discourse of Catastrophe]. (pp. 53–94). Transcript.

Matthewman, S. (2015). *Disasters, Risks and Revelation: Making Sense of Our Times.* Palgrave Macmillan.

McGuire, B. (2012). *Waking the Giant: How a Changing Climate Triggers Earthquakes, Tsunamis, and Volcanoes.* Oxford University Press.

McNeill, W. H. (1976). *Plagues and Peoples.* Anchor Books.

Meding, J. von., Chmutina, K., Forino, G., & Raju, E. (2020). 'Guest Editorial.' *Disaster Prevention and Management 29* (6), 829–30.

Milner, J., Davies, M., Haines, A., Huxley, R., Michie, S., Robertson, L., Siri, J., & Wilkinson, P. (2021). 'Emerging from COVID-19: Lessons for Action on Climate

Change and Health in Cities.' *Journal of Urban Health: Bulletin of the New York Academy of Medicine 98*, 433–437. https://doi.org/10.1007/s11524-020-00501-2.

Montano, S., & Savitt, A. (2020). 'Not All Disasters Are Disasters: Pandemic Categorization and Its Consequences.' *Social Science Research Council*, 10 September. https://items.ssrc.org/covid-19-and-the-social-sciences/disaster-studies/not-all-disasters-are-disasters-pandemic-categorization-and-its-consequences/.

Morens, D. M., & Fauci, A. S. (2020). 'Emerging Pandemic Diseases: How We Got to COVID-19.' *Cell 182* (5), 1077–92.

Nixon, R. (2011). *Slow Violence and the Environmentalism of the Poor*. Harvard University Press.

Oliver-Smith, A. (1999). 'Peru's Five-Hundred-Year Earthquake.' In A. Oliver-Smith, & S. M. Hoffman (Eds.) *The Angry Earth: Disaster in Anthropological Perspective* (pp. 83–93). Routledge.

Patel, S., Webster, R.K., Greenberg, N., Weston, D., & Brooks, S. K. (2020). 'Research Fatigue in COVID-19 Pandemic and Post-Disaster Research: Causes, Consequences and Recommendations.' *Disaster Prevention and Management 29* (4), 445–55.

Penta, S., Kendra, J., Marlowe, V., & Gill, K. (2021). 'A Disaster by Any Other Name? COVID-19 and Support for an All-Hazards Approach.' *Risk, Hazards & Crisis in Public Policy 12* (3), 240-265. https://doi.org/10.1002/rhc3.12213.

Perry, R. (2007). 'What Is a Disaster.' In H. Rodríguez, E. L. Quarantelli, R. R. Dynes, & W. A. Anderson (Eds.) *Handbook of Disaster Research. Handbooks of Sociology and Social Research* (pp. 1–16). Springer Science + Business Media LLC.

Perry, R. W., & Quarantelli, E. L. (Eds.) (2005). *What Is a Disaster? New Answers to Old Questions*. Xlibris.

Pescaroli, G. & Alexander, D. (2015). 'A Definition of Cascading Disasters and Cascading Effects: Going Beyond the "Toppling Dominos" Metaphor.' *Planet@Risk 3* (1). https://planet-risk.org/index.php/pr/article/%20view/208/355.

Prince, S. H. (1920). *Catastrophe and Social Change. Based upon a Sociological Study of the Halifax Disaster*. Columbia University.

Quarantelli, E. L. (1996). 'The Future Is Not the Past Repeated: Projecting Disasters in the 21st Century from Current Trends.' *Journal of Contingencies and Crisis Management 4* (4), 228–41.

Quarantelli, E. L. (2000). *Emergencies, Disaster and Catastrophes Are Different Phenomena*. Preliminary paper #304. Newark, Delaware: Disaster Research Center, University of Delaware.

Quarantelli, E. L. (2005). 'Social Science Research Agenda for the Disasters of the 21st Century: Theoretical, Methodological and Empirical Issues and Their Professional Implementation.' In *What Is a Disaster? New Answers to Old Questions* (pp. 325–96). Xlibris.

Quarantelli, E. L. (Ed.) (2006). *What Is a Disaster? Perspectives on the Question*. Routledge.

Quarantelli, E. L., Lagadec, P., & Boin, A. (2007). 'A Heuristic Approach to Future Disasters and Crises: New, Old, and in-Between Types.' In H. Rodríguez, E. L. Quarantelli, R. R. Dynes, & W. A. Anderson (Eds.) *Handbook of Disaster Research. Handbooks of Sociology and Social Research* (pp. 16–41). Springer Science + Business Media LLC.

Ranghieri, F., & Ishiwatari, M. (2014). *Learning from Megadisasters: Lessons from the Great East Japan Earthquake:* The World Bank.

de Ruiter, M. C., Couasnon, A., Homberg, M. J. C., Daniell, J. E., & Ward, P. J. (2020). 'Why We Can No Longer Ignore Consecutive Disasters.' *Earth's Future 8* (3), 16–25.

de Smet, H., Lagadec, P., & Leysen, J. (2012). 'Disasters Out of the Box: A New Ballgame?' *Journal of Contingencies and Crisis Management 20* (3), 138–48.

Spinney, L. (2017). *Pale Rider: The Spanish Flu of 1918 and How It Changed the World.* Jonathan Cape.

Stallings, R. A. (Ed.) (2002). *Methods of Disaster Research.* Xlibris.

Stallings, R. A., & Quarantelli, E. L. (1985). 'Emergent Citizen Groups and Emergency Management.' *Public Administration Review 45*, 93–100.

Staupe-Delgado, R. (2019). 'Progress, Traditions and Future Directions in Research on Disasters Involving Slow-Onset Hazards.' *Disaster Prevention and Management 28* (5), 623–35.

Tierney, K. J. (2007). 'From the Margins to the Mainstream? Disaster Research at the Crossroads.' *Annual Review of Sociology 33* (1), 503–25.

Tierney, K. J. (2019). *Disasters: A Sociological Approach.* Polity.

Wachira, G. (1997). 'Conflicts in Africa as Compound Disasters: Complex Crises Requiring Comprehensive Responses.' *Journal of Contingencies and Crisis Management 5* (2), 109–17.

Weingärtner, L., & Wilkinson, E. (2019). 'Anticipatory Crisis Financing and Action: Concepts, Initiatives, and Evidence.' *ODI*, 1 July. https://odi.org/en/publications/anticipatory-crisis-financing-and-action-concepts-initiatives-and-evidence/.

Yamori, K., & Goltz, J. D. (2021). 'Disasters Without Borders: The Coronavirus Pandemic, Global Climate Change and the Ascendancy of Gradual Onset Disasters.' *International Journal of Environmental Research and Public Health 18* (6), 3299. https://doi.org/10.3390/ijerph18063299.

7 System rivalry during pandemic times: an institutional political economy view of great power vaccine diplomacy

Naoise McDonagh

Introduction

The COVID-19 pandemic has turbocharged world history while ravaging global populations. From digital transformations of work and education, to the development, clinical testing and distribution of new vaccines in unprecedented timeframes, adapting to the virus has driven structural shifts at breakneck speed viewed historically (see also the chapters by Matthewman and Goode). Perhaps one of the most significant structural shifts the pandemic has accelerated is the growing geopolitical and economic tensions between China and the United States, with some asking whether it marks the end of US hegemony as leader of the post-war liberal international order (Lake et al., 2021; Norrlöf, 2020). Much of the tensions revolve around claims that China's model of state capitalism gives it unfair competitive advantages against liberal capitalist economies. China's trading partners, and most vocally the United States, increasingly argue the country is not meeting its World Trade Organization obligations (Bown & Hillman, 2019; Zhou et al., 2019). Economic competition between the United States and China, in particular, has invoked the view that we are entering a new Cold War type conflict (Karaganov, 2018; Westad, 2019; Zhao, 2019). The pandemic has only added heat to pre-existing tensions, with Bahi arguing: 'The health crisis amplified the competitive dynamics between the USA and China, affected the provision of global public goods[1] and injected instability into the global order' (Bahi, 2021, p. 1). As Goldstein (2020) argues, both countries view the global pandemic as an opportunity and risk to gain or lose influence relative to their competitor.

As economies seek to recover from the economic consequences of the pandemic, trade tensions stemming from different capitalist systems are becoming geopolitical flashpoints that have the potential to intensify and threaten economic recovery (Bahi, 2021). For example, this chapter will assess how growing economic and geopolitical competition is impacting public goods provision through proxy competition between China and the United States, waged as 'vaccine diplomacy' (Zhao, 2021). Provision of vaccines is being used for soft power and influence amongst developing countries in ways that pose both risks and benefits to managing the pandemic. Renewed state-to-state systemic competition between the two largest economies today will have an important effect on the overall ability of the world to combat COVID-19, as well as recover economically from the effects of lockdowns, which in turn impacts future capability to manage health crises. There is a pressing need to understand the nature of these tensions if policies for attenuating Sino-Western tensions are to be devised.

This chapter assesses tension arising from significant ideological and political governance differences between economic models (Evenett, 2021; Wolfe, 2017; Wu, 2016), in a context where China's state capitalist economy has grown to be second largest in the world, a predominant manufacturing power and a direct technological competitor with the United States and Europe. It is suggested that China's historical status as a *returning power* is an important context for understanding China's motives and behaviour in challenging US hegemony in provision of global public goods. Conceptual insights will be drawn from comparative capitalism based on institutional political economy (Boyer, 2005; Deeg & Jackson, 2006; Hodgson, 1996, 2015), which theorizes the role of institutions, culture and history in determining the emergence of variations of capitalism, thus revealing the deep socio-economic roots of today's clash of economic systems. This chapter aims to provide insight into the historical and institutional factors driving this clash with the hope of addressing geopolitical tensions in constructive ways. It proceeds in four further sections. Section two provides an institutional political economy framework for understanding the interactions of culture, history and politics in shaping developmental trajectories of national capitalisms. Section three turns to key historical institutions influencing China's political economy, including its status as a civilizational state, and its current state governance model, which have flow-on consequences for how it manages vaccine donations. Section four addresses systemic competition and vaccine diplomacy during the COVID-19 pandemic. Section five concludes by calling for a research agenda on global cooperation for public goods provision.

Theorizing the persistence of capitalist variation

Institutional political economy draws on foundations laid by economic sociology in explaining why capitalist variation exists. Swedberg (2003) identifies the antecedents of modern comparative capitalism in the work of sociologist Max Weber, and his typological approach to capitalism(s). Weber's typologies included rational capitalism, political capitalism and traditional commercial capitalism, based on a methodological approach that sought to 'ground the notion of capitalism in the everyday activities of the economy, and to get away from the tendency to see capitalism as a system far beyond the individual' (Swedberg, 2003, p.60). Having reconnected capitalism to the exigencies of everyday life, Weber's second step was to ground the individual in their particular social and historical setting, including the existing social norms and rules that regulate behaviour, whereby 'the economic actor orients his/her behaviour not towards other actors but also towards "orders", which consist of prescribed sets of social action that are enforced in different ways' (Swedberg, 2003, p.60). These prescribed social actions include both formal and informal social rules and expectations, grounded in law and tradition. In foregrounding the regulating effect of social order on agency, Weber made the conceptual link between newly emerging capitalist practices of industrialization, and the pre-existing institutionalized, historically grounded social life of individuals. Weber's point was that pre-existing customs and laws of each nation state would influence the concrete enactment of a particular capitalist social order.

Contemporary institutional political economy has conceptualized Weber's intuition as follows. Modern capitalist economies share core market institutions, but the specific historical and cultural environments unique to each nation state inflect upon how capitalist markets emerge, operate and are regulated. The abstract core elements of capitalism as an economic system include: (1) a legal system supporting private property rights; (2) widespread market-based commodity exchange; (3) widespread private ownership of the means of production; (4) widespread wage labour; (5) a developed financial system and widespread credit availability (Hodgson, 2015, p.259). These institutionalized components must predominate a national economy for it to be classed as a capitalist economy, yet the transition from pre-capitalist to capitalist economy is a historical-evolutionary process of interaction with the existing pre-capitalist institutions. 'Institution' here refers to 'durable systems of established and embedded social rules that structure social interactions' (Hodgson, 2004, p.14), and form the basis for Weber's 'social orders'. The interaction between the universal institutions of capitalism and the concrete pre-existing social system of a given nation state results in a national economy that is both the same as other *capitalist* economies (that is, contains the above five core elements), and *sui generis* in its form of capitalism because of the unique historical path dependencies of each state. This specific national history is congealed within a unique matrix of institutions that express 'the outcome of social and political conflicts that are embedded in a specific society for a given historical period' (Boyer, 2005, p. 548). Consequently, the development of capitalism is not only shaped by market relations, but also by pre-existing non-economic institutions such as political parties, the family, organized religion and civil associations who all have a hand in shaping modern economic relations (Deeg & Jackson, 2006, p. 150; Hodgson, 1996, pp. 386–390).

The role of the past in shaping present institutions is called 'path dependence', and refers to how 'a nation's current and past institutions partially determine the direction of future changes' (Clark, 2016, p. 13). As Mahony points out, the concept refers to more than a claim that 'history matters', but rather, involves identifying key events in institutional formation that have a deterministic effect on the pattern of social evolution that follows the given event (Mahoney, 2000, p. 507). Path dependent processes are crucial to understanding capitalist variation. While there are many differences between American and European capitalism – for example approaches to social welfare and universal healthcare – there are also important similarities and shared cultural and political norms arising from European settlement as the antecedent to the emergence of the American federation. A core similarity relates to their political economic foundations in political liberalism, involving clear legal distinctions around the public and private spheres, the sanctity of private property and shared norms on the role of the state as primarily a market regulator rather than market participant. Thus, while there are differences concerning where exactly to draw the line between public and private, as exhibited by Hall and Soskice's well-known taxonomy of 'liberal market economy' (Anglo-Saxon economies) and 'coordinated market economy' (Western European economies) (Hall & Soskice, 2001), these are differences in degree rather than differences in kind.

The North American and European nations that designed the norms and rules of the post-1945 liberal international trading system shared a core political ideology in political liberalism. The emergence of Asian forms of capitalism has challenged many perceived wisdoms concerning the role of the state in leading economic development (Carney et al., 2009). The general view is that Asian economies tend towards distinct hybrid fusions of market institutional relations that are heavily buttressed and/or circumscribed by forms of state intervention and coordination for national policy goals. Chinese capitalism, in particular, has showcased unique institutional arrangements regarding the extent of state activity within the economy (Chen & Rithmire, 2020; Huang,

2008; Peck & Zhang, 2013; Wu, 2016). Furthermore, unlike other Asian economies, with the brief exception of Japan during the 1980s, China is now systemically central to the global economy, is still growing its economy at a high annual rate and is on track to become the largest economy by the late 2020s, surpassing the nominal Gross Domestic Product of the United States. China's largest trading partners, the United States, EU and Japan are increasingly calling for further reform of China's model of state capitalism (McDonagh & Draper, 2020). Furthermore, the long held view that China's post-1978 economic reforms would eventually lead the country to converge with the West politically and normatively are giving way to the view that China is a revisionist rising power (Johnston, 2019, p. 9). How might China as a rising power affect cooperation between Beijing and Washington with regard to the provision of global public goods? The next section synthesizes studies from the cultural and historical literature on China to provide some insight into the key institutions underpinning the Chinese state, which in turn will inform analysis of patterns of emergent geopolitical competition over the provision of global public goods during the pandemic.

Key institutions of China's state capitalism

China has grown increasingly confident in its economic model, a confidence catalysed by the failure of the Western financial system in 2008.[2] However, as a number of recent studies have argued, China's growing confidence is not only a result of its current status, but also due to the fact that it does not view itself as a rising power to begin with, but a returning power, and this will significantly impact its behaviour in the international system (Jacques, 2009; Schuman, 2020). This history can help inform China's motivations in engaging in vaccine diplomacy during COVID-19, as well as its desire to compete with the United States in the provision of global public goods more generally.

A civilizational state

China is what Jacques describes as a 'civilizational state' (2009, pp. 194–232) with a political philosophy profoundly contrary to political liberalism, and a strong sense of self-identification as a leading state power. China's history as a territory encompassing a people with a shared culture and sense of identity goes back at least 2000 years to the Qin victory at the end of the Warring States period (fifth century BC–221BC), which made possible a major unification of territories and politically separate groupings that resulted in what is today viewed as the political and cartographic consolidation of modern China[3] (Jacques, 2009, p.198). China represents the longest continually existing bounded geography with a related community sharing a political and cultural identity. As Wang Gungwu argues, 'what is quintessentially Chinese is the remarkable sense of continuity that seems to have made the civilization increasingly distinctive over the centuries' (Gungwu, 1991, p.2). Pye states that '[w]hat binds the Chinese together is their sense of culture, race, and civilization, not an identification with the nation as a state' (Pye, 1997, p.209). It is a country where the 'only mode of existence is to relive the past. There is no accepted mechanism within the culture for the Chinese to confront the present without falling back on the inspiration and strength of tradition' (Yongnian, 2004, p.81). For this reason Jacques argues that '[t]here are no other people in the world who are so connected to their past and for whom the past – not so much the recent past but the long-ago past – is so relevant and meaningful' (Jacques, 2009, pp.196–197). This powerful relationship with the past is unsurprising given that China's past was highly illustrious by many measures, not least its position as the central state within the tributary system of state-to-state relations.

The tributary system provided the norms which regulated regional geopolitics and trade in East Asia. While China's regional superiority became increasingly apparent during the Tang era (618–907), its apogee was during the fourteenth and eighteenth centuries (Lee, 2018, p.17). During this period, Confucianism, which is widely accepted as having had significant influence on Chinese political thinking and East Asia more broadly, shaped norms around state-to-state relations (Hu, 2007, p.136). Drawing on Confucian concepts of natural hierarchy determined by innate qualities, the Chinese tributary world order 'was an ethical hierarchy, maintained by the power of the Chinese civilization' (Zhao, 2015, p.964). China's sense of natural hegemony was founded in the fact of 'China being internal, large, and high [culturally] and the barbarians being external, small, and low' (Lien-shengYang quoted in Zhao, 2015, p.963), thus, according to Confucian values, China must lead by virtue of its finer qualities, setting the example of right conduct for others to follow. This contrasts sharply with today's liberal order premised on the Westphalian idea of formal equality between states.

Under the Chinese world order '[a]ll countries arranged themselves hierarchically around the Chinese emperor known as the Son of Heaven (天子)' (Zhao, 2015, p.963). Tributary relations were maintained and reproduced through regular ceremonies and ritual, involving presentation of tributes to the Son of Heaven, but missions also received imperial gifts in turn, and had their expenses paid for once on Chinese territory, as a show of benevolence that incurred substantial cost to China. In return, the tributary system of relations managed trade between China and its bordering neighbours on China's terms, as well as the status and position of physical borders and the hierarchical status of states' relative to China. For tributary states it provided order and stability. China's position within the system was not dependent primarily on physical dominance (Lee, 2018, p. 31) – although nor was military coercion entirely absent – rather, it was an original form of 'soft power' that co-opted as much as coerced its neighbours to generate a Chinese-led hegemony.

China's cultural superiority was further expressed in the fact that invaders who established lasting reigns over the country, such as the Mongols during the twelfth and thirteenth centuries, and the Manchu (1644–1912), were Sinicized, with Gungwu noting that 'in every case the 'foreign' rulers adopted Confucian culture and the Confucian system of governance' (Gungwu, 2000, p. 11). China's world order lasted for centuries, and only began to unravel under the challenge of Western colonial expansionism powered by the technological advantages of industrialization during the nineteenth century, beginning what Chinese political leaders refer to as the 'century of humiliation'. This involved China losing territories such as Macau (to Portugal) and Hong Kong (to the United Kingdom), losing its privileged status as hegemon in a Confucian ethical order of hierarchy and being forced to accede to a Western liberal order based on different cultural, political and moral values. It also involved China facing a world where its cultural status was no longer deemed superior but was rather viewed as inferior by Western powers, a position China had not experienced in its 2000 year history as a state. China's rise today, therefore, is not the rise of a new power, but the return to great power status of a state with a long memory of superpower status, cultural superiority and confidence in its own ways and system of governance.

A Confucian-influenced state

Confucius' (551–479 BC) writings only became influential after his death, but came to dominate Chinese culture for the following 2000 years, with Chinese thinking shaped by 'his arguments and moral precepts, its government informed by his principles, and the Analects became established as the most important book in Chinese history' (Jacques, 2009, p. 198). Under political liberalism, the authority of the state is limited in favour of individual rights and autonomy. Under Confucianism, Chinese political philosophy established a set of norms working in the opposite direction to liberalism, wherein an ethical hierarchy subsumed all lower levels of authority under the writ of the higher authority without formal limit (Pye, 1985, p. 41). Authority figures must maintain their position through right moral conduct and virtuous example. This system of ethical governance is explained by Zhao as follows:

> The Chinese order was thus sustained by a heavy stress on ideological orthodoxy, especially on the idea that adherence to the correct teachings would be manifested in virtuous conduct and would enhance one's authority and influence. Right conduct, according to the proper norms, was to move others by its example. (Zhao, 2015, p. 966)

Hierarchy was viewed as a moral imperative, one that, by its nature, was in opposition to the legal limitations of authority devised by political liberalism, and also in fundamental opposition to popular sovereignty. Chinese elites were historically answerable only to the measure of Confucian ethical norms and right conduct, with those lower on the hierarchy having no role in that assessment in principle. As Jacques explains, 'In the Confucian view, the exclusion of the people from government was regarded as a positive virtue, allowing government officials to be responsive to the ethics and ideals with which they had been inculcated' (Jacques, 2009, p. 207). The Chinese emperor sat in the highest position on the hierarchy, with no formal limits on his power, and was expected to act in the universal interest of the people according to the ascribed Confucian values. In practice, the large territory and population of China meant that the emperor's authority was limited absent the modern communication and social technologies needed to manage such a vast state in real time. Yet, in principle, the emperor's rule was absolute, unlike the limitations on rule under Western liberalism. Some recent examples suggest China's political class is publicly re-adopting Confucian norms of tributary hierarchy as the country's political and economic power grows. Yang Jiechi, China's Foreign Minister, at the 2010 Association of South East Asian Nations (ASEAN) regional forum stated 'China is a big country and other countries are small countries and that is just a fact', as a rebuke of twelve South East Asian nations who raised concerns at China's contentious move to claim sovereignty over most of the South China Sea. Likewise, when Lithuania recently pulled out of a China-led 17+1 forum, an annual summit with Eastern European leaders, the *Global Times*, a Communist Party media outlet, admonished the country by declaring 'Lithuania is not qualified to attack China and this is not the way a small country should act'.[4]

Furthermore, there are significant continuities of Confucian political philosophy in contemporary Chinese Communist Party domestic governance. Chinese politics has traditionally been marked by a supremely sovereign state, wherein 'politics has always been seen as coterminous with government, with little involvement from other elites or the people. This was true during the dynastic Confucian era and has remained the case during the Communist period' (Jacques, 2009, p. 207). Much like the dynastic emperor of the past, the Communist Party is enshrined in Article 1 of China's state constitution as a single-party authoritarian power. Article 1 states: 'The socialist system is the fundamental system of the People's Republic of China. Leadership by the Communist Party of China is the defining feature of socialism with Chinese characteristics'.[5] Furthermore, having suffered a decline in its status during early Communist rule, Confucianism has been explicitly revived by the current Chinese Communist Party regime, with Xi Jinping frequently quoting Confucian classics and using Chinese history to justify and explain state policies (Zhao, 2015, p. 962).

Lastly, under Xi, the Party has sought to develop national pride in Chinese culture and the political system, as expressed by the 2016 document *From 'Three Confidence' to 'Four Confidence'* (从'三个自信'到'四个自信').[6] The Confidence Doctrine is a signature philosophy of Xi Jinping, first announced in tripartite form during the 2012 18th National Congress, and expanded with a fourth element in 2016. It calls for '[s]elf-confidence, theoretical confidence, institutional confidence and cultural confidence'. In essence, it calls for China to be confident in its path of socialism with Chinese characteristics (Brown & Bērziņa-Čerenkova, 2018). In a 2015 speech, President Xi stated, 'We are ready to share our experience and opportunities with other countries and welcome them aboard our development train' (Jinping, 2018, p. 574). This indicates that China no longer views further reform towards a more liberal economic model as its goal, but rather seeks not only to follow its own path, but to develop an alternative global model of state-capitalist development, driving growing tensions between it and leading liberal democracies.

System competition and COVID-19 vaccine diplomacy

Some have called the heightening tension between China and the United States, and increasingly the wider Anglo-Saxon and European democracies, a new Cold War (Karaganov, 2018; Zhao, 2019). In the above analysis of Chinese institutional history, conditions for a Cold War-like geopolitical competition are readily apparent. As China returns as a geopolitical power, its political leaders have increasingly referenced its long history as a great civilization, as well as positioning the country as a model for others to follow. The institutional memory of its tributary status as the Middle Kingdom, Confucian norms and contemporary Marxist–Leninist political institutions provide important insights for understanding China's behaviour. They will increasingly shape the competition between liberal–democratic market economies and China in ways reminiscent of the Cold War. Other parallels with the Cold War era lie in the emergence of proxy conflicts between the United States and China in seeking to gain 'spheres of influence' (Allison, 2020), which was a hallmark of those times.[7] The pandemic has become one such arena for proxy competition. As Bahi notes, the pandemic and ensuing health crisis has heightened the 'competitive dynamics between the USA and China which affected the provision of global public goods'. (Bahi, 2021, p.3). A crucial global good required for ending the COVID-19 health crisis is a cooperative global vaccination campaign, using vaccines with the highest efficacy rate (and see Dare and Kingsbury's chapter). However, geopolitical tensions have instead led to a proxy competition that threatens such cooperation by way of 'vaccine diplomacy' (Karásková & Blablová, 2021; Leigh, 2021; Sharun & Dhama, 2021).

Vaccine diplomacy is defined here as leveraging an ability to produce and distribute vaccines to populations other than a government's own national population in order to achieve political purposes. Currently, there is emerging evidence that suggests a great power competition between the United States and China is influencing the production and distribution of vaccines. Vaccine diplomacy may hold benefits for nations, however, there are also risks. Benefits to this diplomacy include vaccines that have been provided through donations, while Chinese manufacturers are also helping partner countries such as the United Arab Emirates, Egypt and Indonesia to establish their own production capacity (Mardell, 2021). Such actions help China enhance its global status and soft power influence (Karásková & Blablová, 2021). By October 2021 the US Biden administration was reported as having pledged to donate 1.1 billion vaccines by the end of 2022 to mainly lower income countries. By October 2021 data from COVAX, an international initiative aimed at equitable access to COVID-19 vaccines and co-directed by the Vaccine Alliance (GAVI), the Coalition for Epidemic Preparedness Innovations (CEPI) and the World Health Organization, indicated the United States had made good on 190 million of vaccines pledged.[8] COVAX data shows the EU is by far the next biggest donor, at 178 million. For reasons discussed below, China's donations are not through COVAX, thus its donations do not show up in the COVAX database. However, data elsewhere indicates that, by 25 October 2021, China had donated 87 million doses.[9] To the extent that such vaccine diplomacy competition supports greater global access to a critical global public good then the effects are positive.

However, there have also been risks evident in the race to lead vaccine donation. For example, by mid-2021, a total of three Chinese vaccine producers were in operation: Sinovac, CanSino and state-owned giant Sinopharm. While this diversity of supply is also positive, these entities were offering Chinese vaccines on the global market despite reluctance by the responsible Chinese-based producers to release clinical trial data (Mardell, 2021). It was reported in mid-2021 that 200 million doses of Sinopharm's vaccine had been administered worldwide before the state-owned firm finally released interim phase 3 clinical data, but even this data was lacking information on the elderly and vulnerable groups (Pinghui & McCarthy, 2021). Using vaccines prior to such data becoming available is highly risky. Developed countries, including the United States, have thus far refused to approve any vaccines with absent phase 3 clinical data on grounds of efficacy and safety. However, given that a small number of rich countries had secured 60% of world vaccine supply up to April 2021 (Sharun & Dhama, 2021), developing countries desperate to access vaccines have understandably been willing to take risks in a bid to reduce COVID-19 deaths by using vaccines absent full clinical transparency. The willingness of Chinese pharmaceutical firms to distribute vaccines lacking such data is arguably a consequence of the country's governance system in general, which lacks transparency, and contains more leeway for decision making based on political expediency rather than rule-based processes and accountability. Internal political pressure to release a vaccine ahead of or in tandem with the United States, and then to engage in vaccine diplomacy, can be understood in the context of a political shift under Xi Xinping that pushes for China to re-assert itself as a civilizational power.

Alongside non-transparent data for distributed vaccines, there have also been reports that China has used access to its COVID-19 vaccines as a geopolitical carrot to entice countries to switch diplomatic ties from Taiwan to China (Londoño, 2021; Stott et al., 2021). Beijing's 'one-China' principle means nation states must choose between Taiwan and China when establishing formal diplomatic ties, as China will not allow both. As of May 2021 only fifteen nations recognize Taipei over China. Picking off Taiwan's remaining official diplomatic relations is designed to further isolate the nation internationally and incentivize Taiwan's leaders to engage in reunification talks with Beijing. In other cases, it has been claimed that vaccines have been used to shore up foreign support for China's Belt and Road initiative (Biyani & Graham, 2021). More worryingly, an EU European External Action Service report released in April 2021 stated:

> Disinformation around the COVID-19 pandemic, measures taken to contain it and vaccine rollout campaigns continue to be significant . . . Russia and China, in particular, continue to intensively promote their own state-produced vaccines around the world. The so-called 'vaccine diplomacy' follows a zero-sum game logic and is combined with disinformation and manipulation efforts to undermine trust in Western-made vaccines, EU institutions and Western/European vaccination strategies.

Strings-attached vaccine diplomacy coupled with disinformation campaigns to undermine some vaccines has serious negative repercussions for achieving global vaccination. Furthermore, China's desire to donate with conditionality reveals why it has not provided any vaccine donations to COVAX to distribute. COVAX works by pooling donated vaccines and then applying a transparent equity model using population-based proportional allocation for participating countries (Herzog et al., 2021). Donating nations have no say in how COVAX distributes vaccines, and its model ensures governance transparency.

These examples highlight the ways in which a crucial global public good can become caught up in the new geopolitical competition between the United States and China, a conflict grounded in their different economic systems. As Goldstein (2020) argues, both countries view the global pandemic as an opportunity and risk to gain or lose influence relative to their competitor. It is clear that, rather than pooling resources to mass produce the most effective vaccines for the fastest possible global access, China, the United States and others are determined to compete to produce and distribute vaccines separately. This may benefit some countries, yet also holds the risk of vaccines with lower relative efficacy being produced and distributed. Other negatives include the possibility of receiving countries being made subject to conditionality under the duress inflicted by the pandemic.

A research agenda for great power cooperation on global health

Current analysis of the extent and consequences of vaccine diplomacy during the pandemic is an important yet under-researched phenomenon. Furthermore, given that the pandemic continues to severely impact the health of nations during 2021, and new variants of COVID-19 continue to emerge, ongoing vaccine development and boosters will likely be needed for some time to come. Cooperation between the two leading economies and national powers, the United States and China, will be crucial to achieve the most effective and efficient solutions to such global problems. However, a failure to grasp the key underlying institutional factors driving tensions between East and West will make it more difficult to develop cooperation. As argued here, key institutional elements in Chinese society, including its civilizational state history, Confucian norms of authority and hierarchy, are important elements to understand Chinese state behaviour as the nation re-asserts itself on the global stage. While this chapter has sought to provide a portrait of some key institutional elements impacting China's state capitalism, it does not claim to be a comprehensive portrait. China is a vast and complex socio-political entity. There are, of course, more institutional elements beyond those discussed here that have influenced contemporary Chinese political economy in important ways. The goal of this chapter was to address aspects of its great power behaviour that have manifested in relation to the global pandemic and vaccine diplomacy.

In the twenty-first century, where nations are vastly more economically interdependent, vaccine diplomacy has emerged during the pandemic as a proxy for great power competition. This has had positive effects, such as increased access for some countries to free vaccines, but has also incentivized governments to promote less effective vaccines on nationalistic grounds, provide vaccines absent clinical data and in some cases attach conditionality to vaccine access. Vaccine diplomacy has also prevented a pooling of resources to maximize resources, production and distribution, generating negative consequences for global health. Research grounded in institutional political economy can contribute to a research agenda for developing cooperation with China by providing insights into the nature of China's political economy, factors driving the country's political behaviour on the international stage and ways to engage with the country's political leadership constructively. However, the latter can no longer be done in a naïve manner that assumes China is evolving into something like a liberal democracy. Thus research should also outline political, economic and ideological differences that are unlikely to disappear any time soon. Such differences mean ongoing competition is now a structural feature of the international system. During the original Cold War the United States and USSR realized that reducing nuclear weapon stockpiles was a global public good, and initiated Strategic Arms Reduction Treaty (START) talks in 1982. This was a unique and positive moment of cooperation on a key global issue, despite intense overall competition. Further research should look at START as a model for developing vaccine cooperation between the United States and China, as well as a model for cooperation on global goods during future crises, in the context of what today appears as a long road ahead of systemic rivalry.

Notes

1   The International Task Force on Global Public Goods defines them as those which are 'broadly conceived as important to the international community, that for the most part cannot or will not be addressed by individual countries acting alone' (Bahi, 2021, p. 3).
2   A 2019 paper by the State Council Information Office of the People's Republic of China titled 'China and the World in the New Era' reflected that the 2008 financial

crisis solidified China's position as the main stabilizing force and source of demand for the global economy. Available at: http://english.www.gov.cn/archive/whitepaper/201909/27/content_WS5d8d80f9c6d0bcf8c4c142ef.html (accessed 21 May 2021).

3   Jacques notes that historical dating of the origins of modern China arguably could stretch to 3000 years, whereas the CCP inflates this to a historically unsupported figure of 5000 years. Examples are found in 'China and the World in the new Era' (p.3) which begins section one with: 'China is a large country with a 5,000-year-old civilization' or Xi Jinping's 2017 speech to the 19th National CCP Congress, which states: 'With a history of more than 5,000 years, our nation created a splendid civilization'. Available at: http://www.xinhuanet.com/english/special/2017-11/03/c_136725942.htm.

4   'Lithuania risks trouble with geopolitical move: *Global Times* editorial', available at: https://www.globaltimes.cn/page/202105/1224253.shtml (accessed 28 May 2021).

5   Available at: http://english.www.gov.cn/archive/lawsregulations/201911/20/content_WS5ed8856ec6d0b3f0e9499913.html.

6   See Feng Pengzhi (冯鹏志), 7 July 2016. Available at http://theory.people.com.cn/n1/2016/0707/c49150-28532466.html.

7   It should be noted that a large qualitative difference is that today's ideological division coincides with deep economic integration between the East and West that never occurred during the original Cold War, thus the analogy has limitations and today's tensions contain many sui generis elements.

8   Source: Our World in Data, 'How many doses have been donated by each country?' https://ourworldindata.org/covid-vaccinations.

9   Source: Bridge Consulting, China COVID-19 Vaccine Tracker. Available at: https://bridgebeijing.com/our-publications/our-publications-1/china-covid-19-vaccines-tracker/.

References

Allison, G. (2020). The New Spheres of Influence: Sharing the Globe with Other Great Powers. *Foreign Affairs, 99*, 30.

Bahi, R. (2021). The Geopolitics of COVID-19: US-China Rivalry and the Imminent Kindleberger Trap. *Review of Economics and Political Science.*

Biyani, N., & Graham, N. (2021). COVID Vaccines: India and China's New Diplomatic Currency. *New Atlantacist.* Atlantic Council. https://www.atlanticcouncil.org/blogs/new-atlanticist/covid-vaccines-india-and-chinas-new-diplomatic-currency/

Bown, C. P., & Hillman, J. A. (2019). WTO'ing a Resolution to the China Subsidy Problem. *Journal of International Economic Law, 22*(4), 557–78.

Boyer, R. (2005). How and Why Capitalisms Differ. *Economy and Society, 34*(4), 509–57.

Brown, K., & Bērziņa-Čerenkova, U. A. (2018). Ideology in the Era of Xi Jinping. *Journal of Chinese Political Science, 23*(3), 323–39.

Carney, M., Gedajlovic, E., & Yang, X. (2009). Varieties of Asian Capitalism: Toward an Institutional Theory of Asian Enterprise. *Asia Pacific Journal of Management, 26*(3), 361–80.

Chen, H., & Rithmire, M. (2020). The Rise of the Investor State: State Capital in the Chinese Economy. *Studies in Comparative International Development, 55*(3), 257–77. doi:10.1007/s12116-020-09308-3

Clark, B. (2016). *The Evolution of Economic Systems: Varieties of Capitalism in the Global Economy*. New York: Oxford University Press.

Deeg, R., & Jackson, G. (2006). Towards a More Dynamic Theory of Capitalist Variety. *Socio-Economic Review, 5*(1), 149–79.

Evenett, S. J. (2021). Taming the Chinese Dragon: A Promising Cornerstone for Transatlantic Trade Cooperation? *Intereconomics, 56*(1), 8–14.

Goldstein, A. (2020). 'The Pandemic and a Deepening U.S.-China Rivalry'. *Perry World House*. https://global.upenn.edu/perryworldhouse/news/pandemic-and-deepening -us-china-rivalry

Gungwu, W. (1991). *The Chineseness of China: Selected Essays*. Oxford University Press.

Gungwu, W. (2000). *Joining the Modern World: Inside and Outside China*. Singapore University Press.

Hall, P., & Soskice, D. (2001). An Introduction to Varieties of Capitalism. In P. A. Hall & D. Soskice (Eds.), *Varieties of Capitalism: The Institutional Foundations of Comparative Advantage* (pp. 1–68). Oxford University Press.

Herzog, L. M., Norheim, O. F., Emanuel, E. J., & McCoy, M. S. (2021). Covax Must go Beyond Proportional Allocation of Covid Vaccines to Ensure Fair and Equitable Access. *British Medical Journal, 372*, 1–3.

Hodgson, G. M. (1996). Varieties of Capitalism and Varieties of Economic Theory. *Review of International Political Economy, 3*(3), 380–433.

Hodgson, G. M. (2004). *The Evolution of Institutional Economics: Agency, Structure and Darwinianism in American Institutionalism*. Routledge.

Hodgson, G. M. (2015). *Conceptualizing Capitalism: Institutions, Evolution, Future*. University of Chicago Press.

Hu, S. (2007). Confucianism and Contemporary Chinese Politics. *Politics & Policy, 35*(1), 136–53.

Huang, Y. (2008). *Capitalism with Chinese Characteristics: Entrepreneurship and the State*. Cambridge University Press.

Jacques, M. (2009). *When China Rules the World: The Rise of the Middle Kingdom and the End of the Western World*. Allen Lane.

Jinping, X. (2018). *Xi Xinping: The Governance of China* (Vol. 2). BetterLink Press Incorporated.

Johnston, A. I. (2019). China in a World of Orders: Rethinking Compliance and Challenge in Beijing's International Relations. *International Security, 44*(2), 9–60.

Karaganov, S. (2018). The New Cold War and the Emerging Greater Eurasia. *Journal of Eurasian Studies, 9*(2), 85–93.

Karásková, I., & Blablová, V. (2021). The Logic of China's Vaccine Diplomacy. *The Diplomat*. 24 March. Retrieved from https://thediplomat.com/2021/03/the -logic-of-chinas-vaccine-diplomacy/

Lake, D. A., Martin, L. L., & Risse, T. (2021). Challenges to the Liberal Order: Reflections on International Organization. *International Organization, 75*(2), 225–57.

Lee, J.-Y. (2018). *China's Hegemony: Four Hundred Years of East Asian Domination by Ji-Young Lee*. Columbia University Press.

Leigh, M. (2021). Vaccine Diplomacy: Soft Power Lessons from China and Russia? *Bruegel*. https://www.bruegel.org/2021/04/vaccine-diplomacy-soft-power -lessons-from-china-and-russia/

Londoño, E. (2021). Paraguay's 'Life and Death' Covid Crisis Gives China Diplomatic Opening. *New York Times*. 16 April. https://www.nytimes.com/2021/04/16/world /americas/paraguay-china-vaccine-diplomacy.html

Mahoney, J. (2000). Path Dependence in Historical Sociology. *Theory and Society, 29*(4), 507–48.

Mardell, J. (2021). Europe Shouldn't Underestimate the Global Appeal of China's Vaccine Diplomacy. *MERICS: Mercator Institute for China Studies.* 3 May. Retrieved from https://merics.org/en/short-analysis/europe-shouldnt -underestimate-global-appeal-chinas-vaccine-diplomacy

McDonagh, N., & Draper, P. (2020). Industrial Subsidies, State-Owned Enterprises and WTO Reform: Prospects for Cooperation? *Institute for Industrial Trade.* 2 September. https://iit.adelaide.edu.au/news/list/2020/09/02/industrial -subsidies-state-owned-enterprises-and-wto-reform-prospects-for

Norrlöf, C. (2020). Is COVID-19 the End of US Hegemony? Public Bads, Leadership Failures and Monetary Hegemony. *International Affairs, 96*(5), 1281–303.

Peck, J., & Zhang, J. (2013). A Variety of Capitalism . . . with Chinese Characteristics? *Journal of Economic Geography, 13*(3), 357–96.

Pinghui, Z., & McCarthy, S. (2021). Chinese Drug Firm Sinopharm Finally Publishes Covid-19 Vaccine Trial Data. *South China Morning Post.* 27 May. https:// www.scmp.com/news/china/science/article/3135067/chinese-drug-firm-sinopharm -finally-publishes-covid-19-vaccine

Pye, L. W. (1985). *Asian Power and Politics: The Cultural Dimensions of Authority.* Harvard University Press.

Pye, L. W. (1997). Chinese Democracy and Constitutional Development. In F. Itoh (Ed.), *China in the Twenty-First Century: Politics, Economy, and Society* (pp. 205–18). United Nations University.

Schuman, M. (2020). *Superpower Interrupted: The Chinese History of the World.* Public Affairs.

Sharun, K., & Dhama, K. (2021). COVID-19 Vaccine Diplomacy and Equitable Access to Vaccines Amid Ongoing Pandemic. *Archives of Medical Research, 52*(7), 761–3.

Stott, M., Hille, K., & Sevastopulo, D. (2021). US to send vaccines to Latin America after Taiwan ally warns of pivot to China. *Financial Times.* May 19. https://www.ft.com /content/c0717932-0d88-4cea-b55c-ff561ed1f70e

Swedberg, R. (2003). *Principles of Economic Sociology.* Princeton, NJ: Princeton University Press.

Westad, O. A. (2019). The sources of Chinese conduct: Are Washington and Beijing fighting a new Cold War. *Foreign Affairs, 98*, 86–95.

Wolfe, R. (2017). Sunshine over Shanghai: Can the WTO illuminate the murky world of Chinese SOEs? *World Trade Review, 16*(4), 713–32.

Wu, M. (2016). The "China, Inc." Challenge to Global Trade Governance. *Harvard International Law Journal, 57*, 261.

Yongnian, Z. (Ed.) (2004). *Will China become democratic? Elite, class and regime transition.* Singapore: Eastern Universities Press.

Zhao, M. (2019). Is a new Cold War inevitable? Chinese perspectives on US–China strategic competition. *The Chinese Journal of International Politics, 12*(3), 371–94.

Zhao, S. (2015). Rethinking the Chinese world order: The imperial cycle and the rise of China. *Journal of contemporary China, 24*(96), 961–82.

Zhao, S. (2021). Why China's vaccine diplomacy is winning. *East Asia Forum.* April 29.

Zhou, W., Gao, H., & Bai, X. (2019). Building a market economy through wto-inspired reform of state-owned enterprises in China. *International & Comparative Law Quarterly, 68*(4), 977–1022.

8   COVID passports: discrimination, inequality and coercion

Tim Dare and Justine Kingsbury

Introduction

The COVID-19 pandemic has prompted extraordinarily intrusive, demanding and expensive lockdowns. As effective COVID-19 vaccines have become available, vaccine passports have come to be seen as key elements of lockdown exit strategies. They contribute to those strategies in at least two ways. First, on the assumptions that they provide reliable evidence of vaccination status, and that vaccination significantly reduces an individual's propensity to contract and to transmit COVID-19 and the severity of the illness if they do catch it, decision makers – from border and health authorities to those controlling entry to nightclubs and football games – have used or are proposing to use them to inform decisions about who may re-engage with others. Second, given that the return to normalcy they allow is attractive to individuals, vaccine passports have been seen as incentives to vaccinate, and so as helping to secure the benefits of increased vaccination rates for individuals and communities. So understood, vaccination passports are attractive, but they have attracted a slew of criticisms, including concerns about whether vaccine passports are discriminatory given the unequal access to vaccines, and the role of passports as vaccination incentives.

In this chapter, we focus on these last two connected issues, arguing that, while the common case against vaccine passports based upon inequality of vaccine access is tempting, there are reasons to treat it with care (Lambert's chapter discusses structural inequities in the health system and McDonagh's chapter discusses great power vaccine diplomacy). One reason to treat the argument with care is that, even if vaccine passports are available unequally, they may incentivise vaccination in ways which improve the position of even those who do not or cannot have access to vaccines and so to vaccine passports. However, vaccine incentives raise ethical problems of their own.[1] If not having a vaccine passport prevents people from earning a living and engaging in other activities crucial to their security and wellbeing, rather than only to 'discretionary' goods and services – restaurant meals, concerts and international travel, for instance – they seem almost certain to run afoul of a coercion objection to incentives, and to do so in ways which are discriminatory and inegalitarian. Most governments have been wary of mandating vaccination, both before and during the COVID-19 pandemic, but it is difficult to reconcile that wariness with the now common willingness to adopt coercive vaccine incentives in the form of vaccination passports. Governments could address these issues by avoiding coercive and discriminatory uses of vaccine passports or by acknowledging that they take COVID-19 to justify coercion and making COVID-19 vaccination compulsory. The latter may be less discriminatory and more candid.

Vaccination passports and inequality of access to vaccines

A central concern about vaccination passports has been the worry that they will cause or exacerbate inequality. One reason to think they might do so is because access to them relies upon access to vaccines and access to vaccines has been unequal.[2] The citizens of some countries are more likely to have access to vaccines – and so to vaccine passports – than the citizens of other countries, and within countries, some individuals and groups are more likely to have access to vaccines than others. Furthermore, these inequalities track familiar and ethically troubling fault lines.

Countries and regions with the highest incomes are getting vaccinated more than thirty times faster than those with the lowest (Randall, 2021). These differences are due in part to differences between the health infrastructures of wealthy and poor countries – itself a legitimate matter for ethical concern – and also to more immediate, explicit and obviously ethically troubling conduct. By late 2020, before the widespread release of vaccines, the governments of high-income countries containing just under fourteen per cent of the world's population had entered into contracts reserving fifty-one per cent of doses proposed for manufacture. Japan, Australia and Canada had reserved more than a billion doses, although they had had less than one per cent of COVID-19 cases (So & Woo, 2020, p. 1). More recently, some wealthy countries have sought to secure supplies for booster shots, notwithstanding that evidence for their benefit is at this point unclear and the concern that if they succeed it will be harder still for poorer countries to vaccinate their citizens at all: 'It would be selfish', said the World Health Organization, 'to give booster doses when so many haven't even had one dose' (Wilkinson et al., 2021).

Within countries, social disadvantage is an important influence on immunisation coverage (Nowlan et al., 2019, p. 80). The poor have always been among those least likely to be vaccinated – they face practical barriers to accessing and using health services, they are more likely to mistrust health systems and so are more prone to vaccination hesitancy – and, typically, ethnic minorities are similarly positioned (in part, no doubt, because they are also more likely to be poor than the members of ethnic majorities). In New Zealand, Māori are being vaccinated at a rate nearly half of that of New Zealanders of European descent despite expert advice that they are at higher risk of infection and adverse outcomes (Neilson, 2021; and see Lambert's chapter and Wyver's contribution for more on the connections between race/ethnicity and COVID-19). The same patterns appear around the world: the Roma community in Hungary, black people in the United Kingdom and the United States, and the Bedouin community in the south of Israel, all identified as at-risk groups, are all vaccinated at a lower rate than the majority communities of their countries (Ganty, 2021, pp. 346–347). 'If vaccination programmes are to protect the whole population, including the poor', writes Sarah Ganty, 'the system of vaccination certificates itself is exclusionary, because of its difficult access for the least socioeconomically privileged people who will not be able to return to pre-pandemic life' (Ganty, 2021, p. 344).

Inequality of access to vaccines is not always morally problematic. There are contra-indicators for COVID-19 vaccines, as there are for all medicines; some people should not have the vaccine on health grounds. The numbers of people who will be unable to be vaccinated on health grounds seems likely to be low. The list of contraindicators for the main COVID vaccines is short. Only those who had experienced an allergic reaction to the first dose of a vaccine itself, or had previously had reactions to any of its components, are now identified as people who should not receive it. Nonetheless, like those who cannot obtain the vaccine because of a lack of access, those who cannot have the vaccine on health grounds will also be unable to obtain a vaccine passport.

The case against vaccine passports based upon inequality of vaccine access is, at least initially, tempting. Vaccine passports are portrayed as compounding the underlying inequality of access; they allow those who have unjustified priority of access to vaccines to cash in on their good fortune. 'Until everyone is able to easily get vaccinated', concludes one vaccine passport critic, 'using vaccine passports to restrict travel and access to spaces can reinforce a system of inequality, deepening discrimination against the less privileged' (Li, 2021).

There are, however, reasons to treat this initial conclusion with care. Imagine the case from the other perspective. Lockdowns involve the significant restriction of a range of important liberties; the liberties to associate with others; to move freely within a country, and so on. Those restrictions are most obviously justified by the important public interest in containing COVID-19. The virus poses very significant health risks and lockdowns are one of the few options for preventing its spread. However, assuming vaccination works – significantly reducing the likelihood that an individual will contract or transmit the virus, and the severity of the illness if they do – then this plausible justification for removing default liberties does not seem to justify restricting liberty of those who have been vaccinated. They pose a relatively low risk of contracting or spreading infection. Absent the extraordinary 'COVID justification' for continuing to curtail their liberties, they should have access to their default liberties. From this perspective, the justification for curtailing liberties has gone; so the curtailment should go too. What requires justification, from this perspective, is the curtailment of default liberties, rather than their restoration.

There also seems to be reason to doubt the claim that introducing vaccine passports despite continuing vaccine access inequality is improperly discriminatory. The modifier 'improperly' is important: discrimination is not improper *per se*. We are permitted, perhaps even required, to discriminate between people on the basis of legitimate differences. We should not treat people with whom we engage as though there were not important and relevant differences between them, and there are relevant and important differences between those who have been vaccinated against COVID-19 and those who have not. The latter are more likely than the former to contract the virus, to suffer more severe symptoms if they do and to transmit the virus to others (Swan et al., 2021). Those differences are relevant to decisions about restricting the liberties of people to travel and to engage with others in communities under threat from the COVID-19 virus. Distinguishing between people on the basis of their COVID immunity may be discrimination, but it is not obvious that is improper, or unjustified, discrimination.

Nonetheless, this discrimination may still be damaging. Allowing the vaccinated to take advantage of their immunity status may 'reinforce a system of inequality', 'deepening' the inequality which provides that advantage in the first place (Li, 2021). As noted, access to vaccines is likely to track familiar distributions of social advantage: those who are better off, better educated, more securely employed, who are members of favoured social groups and so on, are also more likely to have access to vaccines, and so to vaccine passports. It seems plausible that existing gaps between socially advantaged and socially disadvantaged groups will grow if the members of socially advantaged groups can use vaccine passports to return to something approaching their pre-pandemic lives while those who are already disadvantaged cannot. Those with access to vaccines and consequently vaccine passports will be able to return to the productive (and the non-productive) aspects of their lives, increasing their wealth relative to those relying on social support or their own resources. Unequal access to vaccine passports may well 'reinforce' and 'deepen' existing inequalities,[3] widening the existing gap between the antecedently advantaged and disadvantaged.

Again, however, there is another side to this coin. Famously, John Rawls argued that social and economic inequalities should be tolerated only where those inequalities benefit the worst off members of society (Rawls, 1972, p. 302).[4] We might tolerate inequality of income, for instance, if satisfied both that only the promise of significant income led people to train as medical professionals and that the presence of medical professionals benefited the worst off members of our community.[5] The 'difference principle' is premised in part on a rejection of a principle of absolute equality, according to which every person should have the same level of material goods and services. This absolute principle seems to entail that an arrangement in which everyone is equal (arrangement1) is to be preferred over a world (arrangement2) in which everyone is better off than they are in arrangement1, but in which some people are better off than others. Rawls rejects this conclusion. He values equality, but not absolutely. We should tolerate the inequality in arrangement2 if it improves the position of the worst off. We certainly should not 'level down' to arrangement1 from arrangement2 simply to secure equality. It seems plausible that providing vaccine passports to those who have been vaccinated, and by doing so allowing them to return to many or all of their pre-pandemic activities, might improve the position of those who are unable to access vaccines. Those with access to passports, we might suppose, will contribute to the financial and social economy directly through their work, perhaps providing goods and services to those unable to exit lockdown, and through the taxes they pay helping governments provide support to those who for their own sake and the sake of others cannot safely emerge from lockdown. We might appeal to something like the difference principle, that is, to justify unequal access to vaccine passports. That inequality improves the absolute position of those who do not or cannot have access to vaccines, and so to vaccine passports, despite making their relative position worse.

Issuing vaccine passports, even in the face of unequal access to vaccines, may help the unvaccinated in other ways too. Access to vaccine passports is often seen as an incentive to vaccinate. Those who would otherwise not vaccinate, either because they have a positive preference not to, or simply because they fail to get around to doing so, are provided with a reason to do so. Vaccination incentives raise their own issues of discrimination and equality, and we turn to those issues in the next section. For now, on the assumption that it is best for everyone, perhaps especially those who are not vaccinated, if vaccination rates are as high as possible, since high vaccination rates reduce the risk of disease outbreaks which might be especially threatening to the unvaccinated, providing effective incentives to vaccinate is a benefit to the unvaccinated, no matter why they are unvaccinated.[6]

The suggestion so far, then, is that, while the case against vaccine passports based upon inequality of vaccine access is tempting, there are reasons to treat it with care. In sum, we might view vaccine passports as a way of restoring default liberties the curtailment of which is no longer justified once an individual is vaccinated; we might think that even if there is discrimination, that discrimination is not improper since it is based on genuine and relevant differences between the vaccinated and the unvaccinated; and we might think that, even if vaccine passports contribute to ongoing, and perhaps even increasing inequality, that inequality is justified because it improves the position of those who do not or cannot have access to vaccines and so to vaccine passports.

Discrimination, inequality and vaccine incentives

We have appealed to the potential for vaccine passports to incentivise vaccination as part of a response to concerns that COVID vaccination passports may be improperly discriminatory. It has seemed to some, however, that using vaccine passports as incentives is itself discriminatory and inegalitarian (Hart, 2021), since they incentivise unevenly and in ways which, again, track familiar and ethically troubling fault lines; they have more force, and may even be coercive, for those whose resources leave them with few options. We see exactly this effect in other vaccine incentive programmes. The Australian government withholds three significant state payments from parents who fail to vaccinate their children. Prior to 2015, families identifying as conscientious objectors were exempt from these requirements: they could receive the same benefits without having their children vaccinated. The removal of that exemption under the *No Jab No Pay* policy has been linked to vaccine coverage increases of between 2 per cent and 3.8 per cent across the various Australian states (Li & Toll, 2021, pp. 4–5).[7] The results suggest that vaccine incentives work, at least in the sense that they increase vaccination, but our current concerns about discrimination and inequality arise because the increase in vaccination uptake following the removal of the conscientious objection exemptions was, as the Australian researchers put it, 'heterogeneous':

> The improvement in coverage was largest in areas with greater socioeconomic disadvantage, lower median income, more benefit dependency, and higher pre-policy baseline coverage. Overall, while immunisation coverage has increased post removal of conscientious objection, the policies have disproportionally affected lower income families whereas socioeconomically advantaged areas with lower baseline coverage were less responsive. (Li & Toll, 2021, p. 1)

There seems reason to think, then, that the autonomy objection raises genuine concerns: incentives work but they work unevenly. The objection posts a challenge to the use of vaccine passports as vaccine incentives. We need to see whether and how vaccine passports can be used as incentives without being improperly discriminatory or objectionably inegalitarian.

It is useful to begin by considering incentives more generally. An incentive is something offered to alter the utility calculation bearing upon a person's (or community or group's) choice about what to do. The person or agency offering the incentive intends to make an option they prefer more attractive to the person responding to the incentive.[8] The 'autonomy' objection to incentives is that they may overbear the offeree's will. An incentive may be an offer the offeree cannot refuse; it may, that is to say, be coercive. As a conceptual matter, it seems clear that there are coercive incentives. An offer of water might be irresistible to anyone sufficiently dehydrated. We would doubt that their agreement to do something in return for water was freely given. It seems equally clear, however, that there are non-coercive incentives; incentives which operate below the level of inducement at which they pose a threat to autonomy. We all make decisions based on our assessment of the weight of reasons for and against alternatives, and it is rational to prefer options which satisfy our preferences to a greater degree. Our view of incentives cannot entail that all such choices are coerced. Such a position would itself threaten autonomy, refusing to count as autonomous choices freely judged by those making them to be rational and preferable to available alternatives. A plausible and practical approach seems to be to ask whether a reasonable person in the position of the offeree could resist an incentive: if they can do so, they retain the opportunity to act autonomously (whatever they in fact choose to do). The question will never be entirely straightforward – there will be a vast range of offerees and circumstances – but it provides a plausible (or reasonable) test of whether an incentive is coercive.[9]

When thinking about vaccine incentives from this perspective, it is useful to distinguish between those who have strong or principled objections to vaccination and those who have no such objections but who have not been vaccinated for a range of pragmatic reasons: they may be busy; they may not think there is any reason for them to be vaccinated now rather than later; they may think it would be better to be vaccinated later since the vaccine rollout will continue to produce evidence about vaccine safety and efficacy.[10] Call the latter group 'casually' vaccine hesitant.[11] This distinction can be used to design non-coercive incentives (Dare, 2014, pp. 50–6). We remarked that incentives can operate below a level of inducement at which they pose a threat to autonomy. It seems especially plausible that they will do so where they aim to provide a motive to perform an action to which an offeree is not antecedently strongly opposed. If someone's calculation of the utility of vaccination is fairly evenly balanced, perhaps because their inaction is largely due to the sorts of pragmatic reasons sketched above – because that is to say, they are only 'casually' vaccine hesitant – it may not take much to tip the balance in favour of vaccination. If we wish to incentivise vaccinations while minimising the risk that our incentive will be vulnerable to the autonomy objection, we can offer incentives just sufficient to motivate the merely vaccine hesitant. Such incentives are unlikely to motivate those whose calculation of the utility of vaccination is more strongly weighted against vaccination; it is likely they will be able to resist the motivation.

If we wish to use incentives and reduce the risk of running afoul of the coercion objection, then, we ought to avoid targeting the strongly vaccine hesitant, the group who are most likely to require autonomy threatening incentives to overcome their disinclination to vaccinate. So stated, that is an ethical or normative recommendation: we *ought* to pitch incentives at a level at which they do not attempt to motivate the strongly vaccine hesitant. There are empirical, epidemiological reasons to think that we *can* limit the scope of incentives in this way too, at least in the sense that doing so would not make vaccination programmes ineffective. No community needs everyone to be vaccinated. The percentage of a population that must be immune (through vaccination or other means, such as having had and recovered from a vaccine preventable disease) depends upon, inter alia, the basic reproduction number (R_0) of the virus; R_0 is the average number of secondary cases that a primary case will generate in a population in which nobody is either immune or vaccinated. An R_0 value of greater than 1 implies an exponential growth in the number of cases in a population: 100 people with the disease will pass it on to more than 100 other people, who will in turn pass it on to an even larger number of people and so on. An R_0 value below 1 indicates that each person with the disease will, on average, pass it to less than one other person. Epidemics stop once the R_0 value for a virus in a population is smaller than 1. Given an R_0 value below 1, the proportion of the population with the disease will reduce as fewer people have it to pass to others. Importantly, the R_0 value of a virus allows health officials to calculate the immunity or vaccination rate required in a population to stop epidemics. Early estimates of the R_0 for COVID-19 were based on Chinese data (Alimohamadi et al., 2020, p. 155) and reported an estimated R_0 of 3, indicating that the proportion of immune persons needed to stop the outbreak in China would be close to 70 per cent.[12] Note the implication that the COVID-19 epidemic in China would have petered out if even as many as 30 per cent of the Chinese population had remained vulnerable to COVID-19: an R_0 of 3 meant that getting the R_0 level below 1 required only 70 per cent of the population to be vaccination or to have acquired immunity by other means. Further, the value of R_0 is not entirely determined by biological characteristics of the disease. In addition to the (average) number of days that an infected person is contagious (a biological characteristic) it also depends upon the (average) number of daily contacts one contagious person has (the factor targeted by lockdowns) and the probability of transmission of the disease during such a contact. These last two factors are heavily dependent on the social practices of a given community (Delamater et al., 2019, p. 2). Differences in such practices led some researchers to suggest that the R_0 of COVID-19 in Western Europe was significantly lower than that in China, and that consequently the proportion of immune persons in the European population required to stop the outbreak could thus be closer to 50 per cent than to 70 per cent (Locatelli et al., 2021, p. 7). Note the implication that the COVID-19 epidemic in Western Europe would end even if up to 50 per cent of the population remained vulnerable to COVID-19.[13]

This discussion of the R_0 of COVID-19 is relevant to incentives and the autonomy objection to them because, depending on the rate of strongly vaccine hesitant members of a population, it suggests that vaccine incentives need not target the strongly vaccine hesitant, the group who are most likely to require autonomy threatening incentives to overcome their disinclination to vaccinate. All things being equal, we might deliberately set out to provide incentives at a level we would not expect to override the strongly held views of principled anti-vaccinators. We will not mind if the strongly opposed are not amenable to vaccination incentives.[14]

Remember that we are interested in ways to reduce the likelihood that vaccine incentives, and so vaccine passports as incentives, will be vulnerable to the autonomy objection to incentives. An important way to reduce the likelihood that vaccine incentives will do so is to provide support to those individuals in communities we wish to protect from the effects of incentives. Those who have medical contraindications to vaccination are the easy case. Communities should ensure, insofar as they are able, that those who should not be vaccinated on medical grounds are not led to do so by inducements they cannot resist. A choice to vaccinate despite sufficiently serious contraindications may be presumptive evidence of compulsion. One fairly straightforward way to cancel out the effect of incentives on such individuals is to make benefits equal to the value of the incentives available to them without vaccination: many countries which employ vaccine incentives do precisely that.[15] The decision to provide such benefits should be made easier by the fact, as noted, that communities do not need everyone to vaccinate: indeed, one important reason for those able to vaccinate to do so is to protect those who cannot.

Those who choose not to vaccinate on principled, as opposed to medical, grounds are a more challenging case (Clarke et al., 2017). We have seen that Australia and California removed exemptions from incentive programmes which extended benefits to conscientious objectors and that vaccination rates increased in response (Bednarczyk et al., 2019, p. 183; Li & Toll, 2021, pp. 4–5). There is at least one respect in which it is hard to know what to make of these results in light of the previous discussion. With the coercion objection to vaccine incentives in mind, we have suggested, one should pitch incentives at a level at which they are likely to factor in the autonomous reasoning of the 'casually' vaccine hesitant, while not being sufficient to override the autonomy of those who are strongly hesitant. Targeting the latter group with incentives makes it more likely, we think, that incentives will be coercive, simply because we have antecedent reason to think that they have made an autonomous choice not to vaccinate. We have suggested that one way to reduce that risk is to make alternative support available for those who should be able resist incentives. The Australian and Californian results suggest that at least some non-vaccinators did not persist in their choice not to vaccinate once the incentive was applied to them, however, without further research we cannot know whether those who vaccinated their children in response to the loss of the exemption from the incentives were strongly or casually vaccine hesitant.

We have already noted that the Australian and Californian results do show a connection to our earlier concerns about discrimination: 'Overall, while immunisation coverage has increased [in Australia] post removal of conscientious objection, the policies have disproportionally affected lower income families whereas socioeconomically advantaged areas with lower baseline coverage were less responsive' (Li & Toll, 2021, p. 1). These results are not surprising, but they do raise concerns about coercion. If there is any reason to think differences in vaccine hesitancy track socioeconomic advantage, it is likely to increase with social disadvantage. We would expect the poor to be more resistant to vaccination than the well off. As noted, the poor have always been among those least likely to be vaccinated: they face practical barriers to accessing and using health services; they may have less discretionary time to organise vaccinations and they are also more likely to mistrust health systems and so take themselves to have reason to choose not to vaccinate. Their tendency to be more responsive to incentives than those who are better off, given that their baseline vaccine hesitancy is likely to be higher, plausibly shows that they feel they have less choice: they need the incentives and so can be coerced by them. The incentives are an offer they cannot refuse.

We have suggested pitching incentives at levels such that reasonable offerees can decline them. The discussion has ranged over vaccine incentives in general and vaccine passports as incentives in particular. There is a further point of particular relevance to COVID-19 vaccination passports to be made here. The purpose for which vaccination passports are or are not intended to be used is central to their ethical evaluation: it matters just what they are passports to. Under some proposals, COVID-19 vaccination passports are essentially travel documents, like the eponymous passports from which they take their name, to be used with them at the same decision points, allowing airlines or border control authorities to verify the vaccination and COVID-19 health status of would-be travellers.[16] It is easy to see why this use is attractive: international travel is undoubtedly important to many individuals, to the international travel industry and to economies more generally; controlling international borders has been central to many countries' COVID-19 strategies; furthermore, freedom of movement may be regarded as important in its own right, independently of its tendency to promote economic or other desirable goals.[17]

Nonetheless, for most of the world's population international travel is not an everyday and central part of the good life. Bracketing pressing needs to escape unsafe situations arising from war or famine – or plague – most people most of the time are not significantly disadvantaged by limitations on international travel. Increasingly, however, countries are proposing to use, or are using, vaccine passports more broadly, to control access to a significant, perhaps exhaustive, range of domestic activities.[18] These broad domestic applications are crucial to the role of vaccine passports as vaccine incentives. Since relatively few people are likely to be motivated by the possibility of international travel, relatively few people are likely to be motivated by a vaccination passport which delivers only that benefit. However, the increased incentive value of domestic, broadly applied, vaccine passports raises precisely the concerns we have been discussing. The broader and less discretionary the range of activities controlled or regulated by vaccine passports, the more likely it is that the passport incentive will be coercive, and the more likely it is that that coercion will bear unequally on those who have few alternatives but to return to work and a regular life as soon as possible. If not having a vaccine passport prevents people from earning a living and engaging in other activities crucial to their security and wellbeing, rather than only to 'discretionary' goods and services – restaurant meals, concerts and international travel, for instance – vaccine passports seem almost certain to run afoul of the coercion objection, and to do so in ways which are discriminatory and inegalitarian, posing much greater pressure on those who are already socially disadvantaged.

It might seem that there is an obvious response to these concerns: why worry so much about coercion? Communities are sometimes justified in giving people reasons for action which override their autonomy: the sanctions attached to many laws are intended to do so, for instance, and one might think that the threat posed by COVID-19 warrants a similar approach. It is noteworthy, first, however, that most countries have been wary of directly compelling vaccination both before and during the COVID pandemic. Even as many countries have required workers in some high risk roles to be vaccinated (see for instance *COVID-19 Public Health Response [Vaccinations] Order 2021*), they have explicitly assured the general population that '[i]t will not be mandatory to have the vaccine, which means you won't be required to have it. Having a COVID-19 vaccine is voluntary, which means you can choose whether or not to have it' (Health Navigator New Zealand, 2021). An important part of the explanation for this reluctance is no doubt pragmatic: governments have compelled sparingly and reluctantly, because compulsion is risky. A high level of trust and cooperation has been an important contributor to New Zealand's relative success in controlling COVID-19 and there is well founded apprehension that compulsion would erode those important resources (Vaithianathan et al., 2020).

However, it is hard to reconcile this reluctance, and the probable reasons for it, with proposals to use vaccine passports in ways that impose dramatically and unequally weighted reasons on different portions of populations, and that do so in ways which track and reinforce long recognised social inequities. It is difficult to see, for instance, how New Zealand can consistently introduce vaccine passports in ways which will have those coercive and discriminatory effects, while also announcing that '[h]aving a COVID-19 vaccine is voluntary, which means you can choose whether or not to have it'. For many, especially disadvantaged New Zealanders and their counterparts around that world, that will be false. The incentives posed by wide-ranging domestic vaccine passports will be an offer they cannot refuse. This is a consistency argument, and such arguments always cut both ways: governments could address the issue by avoiding uses of vaccine passports that are coercive, discriminatory and egalitarian, or by acknowledging that they take COVID to justify coercion and making COVID vaccination compulsion explicit. It seems unlikely that taking the latter option would do more harm to trust and cooperation than the surreptitious and uneven compulsion provided by wide-ranging domestic vaccine passports, and it would be less discriminatory.

Notes

1   For discussions around ethics and research, see the contributions by Lambert; Dittmer and Lorenz; Wynn and Trnka; and Southerton, Clark, Watson & Lupton in this collection.
2   Eligibility criteria for vaccine passports vary, and not all rely solely on vaccination. The EU's Green Pass is described as a digital proof that a person has either been vaccinated, received a negative text or recovered from COVID-19 (*EU Digital COVID Certificate*, n.d.). 'Immunity Certificates' – available for those who have contracted and recovered from COVID-19, as opposed to those who have received an approved vaccine or who test negative – raise distinct ethical issues, most obviously by creating perverse incentives to deliberately risk infection. Some uninfected individuals, desperate to obtain a passport, may deliberately risk infection, betting that they will recover, but there are clear risks around such behaviour: individuals might lose that bet, and, in any event, communities are likely to suffer as they spread the virus before recovering or not. Those risks, to both individuals and communities, have increased as deadlier, more transmissible varieties of the virus have emerged.
3   The phenomenon should not be a surprise: inequalities are typically compounding.
4   Rawls deploys the 'difference principle' in a different context, using it to generate basic principles of distributive justice. We do not claim he would have endorsed this application of his influential principle.
5   Of course we might doubt either or both of these assumptions. See, for instance Cohen (1992) and the large literature it inspired.
6   We have not discussed another common defence of vaccine passports, which appeals to earlier and existing requirements for vaccine certification, such as the World Health Organisation's 'Yellow Card', an international certificate recording inoculations against yellow fever, cholera, typhus and smallpox that has been around since the 1930s. The argument, in short, seems to be that we should not object to vaccine passports because we have not objected to the Yellow Card (and they are the same, really): see, for instance, Austracio's contribution in Meaney and Austracio (2021). However, it is not clear what we should make of the example. Perhaps we should have objected to the Yellow Card: it might pose significant ethical risk too; as serious as the Yellow Card diseases are, they are rare or endemic to certain areas: the scale of the COVID-19 pandemic makes some ethical risks more likely and more pressing; some of those risks of vaccine passports (not discussed here) flow from their appearance in a digital age, where information can be held and shared in ways unimaginable only a couple of decades ago; and the Yellow Card has the backing of international health regulations that specify conditions for validity whereas, at the moment at least, COVID passports are being developed independently, by different governments and even by private industries such as the International Air Travel Association (*IATA Travel Pass Initiative*, n.d.).
7   Similar effects were identified in California when the state eliminated personal belief exemption from required vaccinations following a measles outbreak during 2013–15. Although the researchers note various confounders, they suggest that the changes led to an increase in childhood vaccination coverage of nearly 3 per cent in the 2016–17 school year (Bednarczyk et al., 2019, p. 183).
8   We can put aside cases in which incentivisation is problematic because of some feature of the incentivised choice itself; cases in which an incentive is offered to encourage someone to do something illegal or improper or is something which

the offeror ought not encourage the offeree to do. These cases are ethically, and perhaps legally, problematic and they involve incentives, but they are problematic because of the nature of the incentivised choice, not because of some feature of incentives themselves.

9   Elsewhere Dare discussed a more abstract issue around incentives and autonomy. Even accepting that incentives need not be coercive, they may still appear problematic viewed from an ideal standard of 'autonomy respecting discourse' since incentives may seem not to be the *kind* of reason which properly respects the rationality of offerees. In health contexts, we might suppose, for instance, that a rational person should make health decisions on the basis of health reasons. Monetary incentives or the like may provide someone with a reason to vaccinate, but they are not health reasons; they are not relevant to the reasoned assessment of the merits of vaccination, even though they may be relevant to the reasoned assessment of what it is 'best' for an agent to do, all things considered. See Dare (2014, pp. 54–55).

10   And, for the current discussion, putting aside those who do not have access to vaccination or who have health reasons not to vaccinate. Vaccine incentives cannot make a difference to either group, since their vaccine status is not a matter of choice. Perhaps more precisely, incentives cannot make a difference to those who have no access and should not make a difference to those who have health reasons not to vaccinate.

11   In earlier research Dare suggested that most people who failed to have their children vaccinated in New Zealand did so for these sorts of pragmatic reasons, and draws the implication that compulsion was unwarranted, suggesting that very moderate 'nudging' would suffice to change behaviour (Dare, 1998, pp. 137–8).

12   It is important to emphasise that the epidemiological facts matter here (and see Wallace and Wallace in this book). The proportion of a population which can remain unvaccinated without prolonging vaccine preventable disease outbreaks depends on, inter alia, the R_o value of the virus, the efficacy of available vaccines (the lower the percentage of a population who has been vaccinated, the more effective a vaccination must be to deliver the same reduction in the R_0 value [Bartsch et al., 2020, p. 495]); the proportion of the population who cannot be vaccinated, and the proportion of the population who could but will not be vaccinated given some vaccination programme.

13   Note that our argument does not depend on the details of these empirical claims. We are philosophers, not scientists, and in any case the science in this area is fast moving – see Kingsbury and Dare (2017) for suggestions about how to avoid some of the pitfalls of appealing to scientific results as a non-scientist.

14   There may be a practical problem with my practical suggestion to target incentives at the 'merely' vaccine hesitant. A declared 50 per cent vaccination rate might encourage people to think they leave vaccination to someone else, and so might lead to less than 50 per cent coverage. It might be best, that is to say, to incentivise vaccination aimed at getting as close to 100 per cent coverage as possible, knowing that the achieved rate will be some way below that figure.

15   See for instance Australia's *No Jab No Pay* policy, noted earlier and discussed again shortly. It removed exemptions which allowed conscientious objectors to claim benefits equivalent to significant vaccine incentives, but left them in place for those with genuine health reasons to avoid vaccination (Australian Government Department of Health, 2017).

16   See the International Air Travel Association's 'Travel Pass' app, intended to facilitate international flights, and the European Union's Digital Covid

Certificate, introduced in order to restore freedom of movement within Europe (*IATA Travel Pass Initiative*, n.d.; *EU Digital COVID Certificate*, n.d.). Many vaccination passports (the IATA Travel Pass, for instance) vary in an important way from the passports we know best. The value of regular passports rests on the shared international standards that lie behind them. If someone produces a valid NZ passport, an immigration official knows they are a New Zealand citizen, that their identity has been confirmed, that their passport photo is a reasonable likeness, and so on. There are no such shared standards for vaccine passports, so it is much less clear what can be assumed about the passport holder. The very thing that makes passports valuable might not be true of vaccine passports.

17   The importance of the right to freedom of movement is evident in its recognition in a range of international human rights instruments, including the International Covenant on Civil and Political Rights (Articles 12 and 13); the Convention on the Rights of the Child (Article 10); the Convention on the Rights of Persons with Disabilities (Article 18); the Convention on the Elimination of All Forms of Racial Discrimination (Article 5) and the Convention on the Elimination of All Forms of Discrimination Against Women (Article 15).

18   See for instance, Israel's Green Pass, intended from the outset to facilitate participation in wide range of activities, from cultural and sporting events, to gym classes and restaurant dining (*What Is the Green Pass Scheme?*, n.d.; Wilf-Miron et al., 2021) and recent schemes adopted in France and Italy (Hart, 2021) and proposed in New Zealand (Giovannetti, 2021).

References

Alimohamadi, Y., Taghdir, M., & Sepandi, M. (2020). Estimate of the basic reproduction number for COVID-19: A systematic review and meta-analysis. *Journal of Preventive Medicine and Public Health*, *53*(3), 151–7.

Australian Government Department of Health. (2017). (*No Jab No Pay new requirements fact sheet* [Text]). December 18. *Australian Government Department of Health*. https://www.health.gov.au/resources/publications/no-jab-no-pay-new -requirements-fact-sheet

Bartsch, S. M., O'Shea, K. J., Ferguson, M. C., Bottazzi, M. E., Wedlock, P. T., Strych, U., McKinnell, J. A., Siegmund, S. S., Cox, S. N., & Hotez, P. J. (2020). Vaccine efficacy needed for a COVID-19 coronavirus vaccine to prevent or stop an epidemic as the sole intervention. *American Journal of Preventive Medicine*, *59*(4), 493–503.

Bednarczyk, R. A., King, A. R., Lahijani, A., & Omer, S. B. (2019). Current landscape of nonmedical vaccination exemptions in the United States: Impact of policy changes. *Expert Review of Vaccines*, *18*(2), 175–90.

Clarke, S., Giubilini, A., & Walker, M. J. (2017). Conscientious objection to vaccination. *Bioethics*, *31*(3), 155–61.

Cohen, G. A. (1992). Incentives, inequality, and community. *The Tanner Lectures on Human Values*, *13*, 263–329.

COVID-19 Public Health Response (Vaccinations) Order 2021 (LI 2021/94) (as at 12 August 2021) 7 Duty of affected person not to carry out certain work unless vaccinated. New Zealand Legislation. https://www.legislation.govt.nz/regulation /public/2021/0094/latest/LMS487894.html

Dare, T. (1998). Mass immunisation programmes: Some philosophical issues. *Bioethics*, *12*(2), 125–49.

Dare, T. (2014). Disagreement over vaccination programmes: Deep or merely complex and why does it matter? *HEC Forum*, *26*(1), 43–57.

Delamater, P. L., Street, E. J., Leslie, T. F., Yang, Y. T., & Jacobsen, K. H. (2019). Complexity of the basic reproduction number (R0). *Emerging Infectious Diseases*, *25*(1), 1–4.

EU Digital COVID Certificate. (n.d.). [Text]. European Commission – European Commission. https://ec.europa.eu/info/live-work-travel-eu/coronavirus-response /safe-covid-19-vaccines-europeans/eu-digital-covid-certificate_en

Ganty, S. (2021). The veil of the COVID-19 vaccination certificates: Ignorance of poverty, injustice towards the poor. *European Journal of Risk Regulation*, 1–12. Cambridge Core. https://doi.org/10.1017/err.2021.23

Giovannetti, J. (2021). COVID-19 coronavirus Delta outbreak: NZ to have vaccine passport by Christmas. *New Zealand Herald*, 9 September. https://www.nzherald.co.nz/nz /covid-19-coronavirus-delta-outbreak-nz-to-have-vaccine-passport-by-christmas /BWHHR6BDTFXWDXFQOLKCY7KKTI/

Hart, R. (2021). Vaccine passports spur explosion in vaccinations—and protests—as Europe cracks down on vaccine holdouts. *Forbes*, 27 July. https://www.forbes.com /sites/roberthart/2021/07/27/explosion-in-vaccinations-and-protests-follow-health -pass-announcements-as-europe-cracks-down-on-vaccine-holdouts/

Health Navigator New Zealand. (2021). *COVID-19 vaccines | Health Navigator NZ*. Health Navigator New Zealand. https://www.healthnavigator.org.nz/medicines/c /covid-19-vaccines/

IATA Travel Pass Initiative. (n.d.). Retrieved September 11, 2021, from https://www .iata.org/en/programs/passenger/travel-pass/

Kingsbury, J. and Dare, T. (2017). The philosophical use and misuse of science. *Metaphilosophy 48*(4), 449–66.

Li, A., & Toll, M. (2021). Removing conscientious objection: The impact of 'No Jab No Pay' and 'No Jab No Play' vaccine policies in Australia. *Preventive Medicine*, *145*, 106406.

Li, T. (2021). There's a big gaping hole in the plan to issue 'vaccine passports.' *MSNBC.Com*, 23 April. https://www.msnbc.com/opinion/risks-covid-vaccine -passports-are-scarier-you-might-think-n1265023

Locatelli, I., Trächsel, B., & Rousson, V. (2021). Estimating the basic reproduction number for COVID-19 in Western Europe. *Plos One*, *16*(3), e0248731.

Meaney, J., & Austracio, N. (2021). The ethics of COVID-19 vaccine passports. *Ethics & Medics*, *46*(4), 1–2. https://doi.org/10.5840/em20214646

Neilson, M. (2021). COVID-19 coronavirus: Māori vaccination rate nearly half that of Pākehā, Asian populations – 'it's a crisis.' *New Zealand Herald*, 1 July. https://www. nzherald.co.nz/kahu/covid-19-coronavirus-maori-vaccination-rate-nearly-half-that -of-pakeha-asian-populations-its-a-crisis/C36GL72JJEHMHUONBSVEGMV2WQ/

Nowlan, M., Willing, E., & Turner, N. (2019). Influences and policies that affect immunisation coverage—a summary review of literature. *The New Zealand Medical Journal*, *132*(1501), 79–88.

Randall, T. (2021). The world's wealthiest countries are getting vaccinated 25 times faster—Google Search. *Bloomberg Equality*, 9 April. https://www.google.com/search ?q=%27The+World%E2%80%99s+Wealthiest+Countries+Are+Getting+Vaccinated +25+Times+Faster%27&oq=%27The+World%E2%80%99s+Wealthiest+Countries +Are+Getting+Vaccinated+25+Times+Faster%27&aqs=chrome..69i57j0i22i30j69i60 .1780j0j15&sourceid=chrome&ie=UTF-8

Rawls, J. (1972). *A Theory of Justice*. Clarendon Press.

So, A. D., & Woo, J. (2020). Reserving coronavirus disease 2019 vaccines for global access: Cross sectional analysis. *BMJ, 371*.

Swan, D. A., Bracis, C., Janes, H., Moore, M., Matrajt, L., Reeves, D. B., Burns, E., Donnell, D., Cohen, M. S., Schiffer, J. T., & Dimitrov, D. (2021). COVID-19 vaccines that reduce symptoms but do not block infection need higher coverage and faster rollout to achieve population impact. *Scientific Reports, 11*(1), 15531. https://doi .org/10.1038/s41598-021-94719-y

Vaithianathan, R., Ryan, M., Anchugina, N., Selvey, L., Dare, T., & Brown, A. (2020). *Digital contact tracing for COVID-19: A primer for policymakers*. Working Paper.

What Is the Green Pass Scheme? (n.d.). Corona Traffic Light Model (Ramzor). https:// corona.health.gov.il/en/directives/green-pass-info/

Wilf-Miron, R., Myers, V., & Saban, M. (2021). Incentivizing vaccination uptake: The 'Green Pass' proposal in Israel. *JAMA, 325*(15), 1503. https://doi.org/10.1001 /jama.2021.4300

Wilkinson, D., Pugh, J., & Savulescu, J. (2021). COVID: WHO calls for moratorium on booster shots – is it justifiable? *The Conversation*, 17 August. http://theconversation .com/covid-who-calls-for-moratorium-on-booster-shots-is-it-justifiable-165762

9   The care crisis: a research priority for the pandemic era and beyond

Kate Huppatz and Lyn Craig

Introduction

Care has long been identified as being in a state of crisis. Rich nations have been described as experiencing a 'care deficit' in that the demand for care cannot be met by existing relationships and infrastructures (Ehrenreich and Hochschild, 2002, p. 8). This deficit is a direct result of men's unwillingness to engage in unpaid or paid care, women's increased participation in paid labour, aging populations, smaller families and reduced welfare states (Ehrenreich and Hochschild, 2002). This is a crisis that is created in a capitalist system where workers are required to be free of care, without adequate infrastructure for workers to be care free: unfortunately, 'capitalism structurally depends on a fundamental that it cannot create itself' (Livnat and Braslavsky, 2020, p. 272).

These are not ideal conditions from which to respond to a global health crisis. As a consequence, during COVID-19 we have witnessed the amplification of the care deficit alongside, mostly unfulfilled, opportunities for change. The extent to which the care deficit has deepened, has, of course, varied according to local and national context. The acuteness of the COVID-19 care crisis has very much depended upon existing structures, especially welfare and health systems, cultures, geographies, political will and economic resources. As a rule of thumb, however, the longer the lockdowns and childcare and school closures, and the bigger the strain on the healthcare system, the worse the nation's COVID-19 care crisis.

This amplified care crisis has most significantly impacted those who had already been working overtime to fill the care deficit – women (Mooi-Reci and Risman, 2021). Care is a feminised activity, and it is well documented that women do the majority of the unpaid care labour to the detriment of their employment and wellbeing. In response to the loss of childcare and schooling during the pandemic, heterosexual families in particular have adopted, or further invested in, a traditional gendered division of labour, compromising women's economic security and independence (Collins et al., 2021). In the United States, for example, which is one of the few rich nations to fail to provide its citizens with state funded childcare, the closure of childcare centres and limited availability of nannies and babysitters has led to millions of women reducing their paid working hours or leaving employment altogether, in order to address the care shortfall. Thus, the pandemic reveals the gendered dimension to the crisis of care, and how, combined, childcare and schooling are, in fact 'a critical infrastructure of care', that ease the care burden and corresponding inequalities (Collins et al., 2021).

In this chapter we draw upon two broad areas of care research and commentary during COVID-19 – unpaid domestic labour and the employment experiences of academic workers who are carers – to examine 'pinch points' of this crisis; moments where the care deficit has been most apparent or amplified by the coronavirus in households and organisations. This is not a systematic review. Rather it is directed by our own research interests and popular commentary. Nevertheless, our focus on these two areas of research does help us to consider the ramifications of the care deficit for both homes and workplaces, and the ways in which family relationships and organisational cultures might mutually reinforce the care gap. Using these case studies, we make suggestions for a future research agenda for the analysis of the impact of COVID-19 on domestic spaces and the academy, and for the amelioration of the pre-existing and worsening care deficit.

Domestic labour during lockdown

The gendered division of domestic labour has been an enduring phenomenon in households, even as women's workforce participation has increased, and fathers are expected to be more actively involved in child raising (Doucet, 2020). Although most families are now dual earner (Lewis, 2009), women still do significantly more housework and care than men. Notwithstanding some variation by characteristics such as education, earnings, age or attitudes, over time gender has consistently proved the strongest predictor of time in domestic labour and it is usually women, not men, who tailor their paid work patterns around family care needs (Altintas and Sullivan, 2016; Perry-Jenkins and Gerstel, 2020).

Moreover, trying to fit it all in has made households with dependants to care for more and more time pressured. Accounting for the paid and unpaid work of both partners, total household workloads have risen markedly (Craig et al., 2020). There are only 24 hours in the day, and if work and family time demands are too high, something must give. The resulting time scarcity squeezes out time for other activities including sleep, leisure, exercise and socialising, which are necessary to health and wellbeing (Craig and Brown, 2017; Strazdins et al., 2011). Unsurprisingly, there is rising stress, with a fifth of Australian women under 35 diagnosed with depression or anxiety disorders in 2018 (AIHW, 2019; HILDA, 2019). This trend is reflected worldwide. Globally, depression now constitutes 10 per cent of non-fatal disease, and women are twice as likely as men to suffer it (Salk et al., 2017; World Health Organization, 2016). For many families, and particularly women, a care crisis was already manifest in their daily reality before COVID-19 struck.

However, the pandemic lockdowns upturned everyday practice in managing work and care, requiring men and women alike to stay home. Researchers were curious to know whether this would provide opportunity to divide unpaid housework and care labour differently. In their study on divisions of labour in Australia during COVID-19 lockdown, Craig and Churchill found that in households with care-giving responsibilities paid work time was slightly lower, but time in housework and care was very much higher (Craig and Churchill, 2020; 2021a). These time increases were most for women, in line with pre-existing patterns. However, consistent with findings in the United States and the United Kingdom (Carlson et al., 2020; Sevilla and Smith, 2020), gender gaps in care somewhat narrowed because men pitched in more too (Craig and Churchill, 2020; 2021a). The improvement in relative equity was modest, however. As time went on, it became clear that women worldwide were shouldering by far the greater burden of extra housework, home schooling and childcare (Andrew et al., 2020; Collins et al., 2021; Petts et al., 2020; Power, 2020; Schieman et al., 2021).

From a subjective point of view, combining work and family demands during the pandemic was stressful and at times overwhelming for women, many of whom reported a lack of support from their male partners (Craig, 2020). Divisions of labour were more equal in same sex families, but in heterosexual couples there were pervasive implicit or explicit assumptions about women being the default care providers and men's work and careers being more valued and more important (Craig and Churchill, 2021a; 2021b). Men's work commitments took precedence in terms of access to dedicated private workspace as well as time (Craig et al., forthcoming; Skountridaki et al., 2020). This inequity was further compounded by expectations from employers and the workplace. Consistent with pre-existing notions of men as 'ideal workers' unencumbered by care responsibilities (Livnat and Braslavsky, 2020; Williams et al., 2013), most employers seemed to expect that home-based workers would deliver the same output as before the pandemic. The special difficulties of working and caring for children simultaneously in the same physical location were considered by employers as family matters, not requiring workplace support (Craig and Churchill, 2020).

There were negative psychological and emotional consequences of these employer expectations of unaffected productivity, together with gendered domestic inequality (Nieuwenhuis and Yerkes, 2021). By increasing women's housework and childcare beyond a threshold, the pandemic created a wide gender gap in self-rated work productivity and job satisfaction (Feng and Savani, 2021). There was heightened insecurity, with many feeling their jobs were under threat if they could not perform to the level expected (Craig and Churchill, 2020) (social inequalities are also discussed in the chapters by Matthewman; Lambert; and Wyver). Working parents who adapted their work patterns during COVID-19, who were disproportionately women, experienced more psychological distress than those who did not (Xue and McMunn, 2021). A large study across the United States, Canada, Denmark, Brazil and Spain found that, to the extent that women spent more time on tasks such as childcare and household chores than men under lockdown, they reported lower happiness (Giurge et al., 2021).

This is not to say that men were not under pressure too. This showed up in their reports of satisfaction with how domestic work was shared within households. Before the pandemic, less than 10 per cent of men had been dissatisfied with their partners' share of domestic labour and care. During the pandemic, this proportion had more than doubled (Craig and Churchill, 2020). However, men were still doing significantly less unpaid work than women (and no more than women had been doing pre-pandemic), which suggests a relatively low threshold before men feel it is too much, and unfair on them. It could be because employer expectations weighed heavily upon them. The implication is that both employers' and men's own attitudes would need to change substantially if women's careers are not to continue being first to be sacrificed next time a family encounters the pointy end of everyday stressors (Craig et al., forthcoming).

On a more positive note, Craig and Churchill's study showed that, during the pandemic lockdown, many people felt less rushed and pressed for time, due to relief from the daily commute, and from external deadlines including school and day-care drop-offs (Craig and Churchill, 2020; 2021a). This highlights the need for flexibility to support families to organise their daily lives as suits them best. This is both a matter of workplace attitudes and policies, and of how families can maximise their time. In a post-COVID world this means that workplaces should keep allowing employees to work from home when possible, but it also suggests that cutting commuting times through improved transport services would improve daily lives significantly. Also, if women are expected to take on the domestic load by their partners and given no relief from productivity expectations by their employers, they need to rely on non-parental childcare, which again underscores how necessary external care services and infrastructure are to families (Collins et al., 2021).

Academic productivity

Although all industries and organisations differ in their workplace structures and cultures, research on the impact of the pandemic on academic productivity gives some evidence to the consequences of this intensified domestic labour, alongside sustained employment demands, for primary carers. While there has been an amazing output of rapid response research from universities during COVID-19, indicating that many academics are finding space to research and write, there is a gendered pattern to this productivity, with women, especially those with young dependent children, reporting a larger decline in research time than that experienced by men (Myers et al., 2020). In other words, while some academics are 'aiming for the stars' during the pandemic, the high research achievers tend to be those who have less care obligations (Minello, 2020). An issue of significant concern, voiced by those who research gender and academia, has been the disparity between women's and men's publication outputs during the pandemic. This concern was initially sparked by journal editors who observed a reduction in submissions from women in 2020 (see for example, Matthewman and Huppatz, 2020), and has been commented on in higher education research, media and social media (Periera, 2021, p. 3). Some editors claimed that while they witnessed a 20 to 30 per cent increase in submissions, it was men who were increasing their article submissions rather than women (Beck, 2020, cited in Cui et al., 2020). In fact, some journals have reported that men's submissions have increased by up to 50 per cent (Fazackerley, 2020). In perhaps the most comprehensive recent peer reviewed analysis on the impacts of the pandemic on academic publications, Cui and co-authors (2020) found this to be an international trend. Their research, which focused on an open-access pre-print repository for publications in the social sciences, found that, in the United States, in the period from December 2018 to May 2019, in comparison with December 2019 to May 2020, women's publication productivity dropped by 13.2 per cent relative to men's productivity. Across seven countries – the United

States, Japan, China, Australia, Italy, the Netherlands and the United Kingdom – this gender gap was most pronounced for: those at the rank of assistant professor, as this cohort of workers are more likely to be of an age where they have young children and feel pressured to publish; and academics employed at prestigious research universities, as the pressure to produce may be higher in these institutions (Cui et al., 2020).

Therefore, although not all women are mothers or carers, it does appear that, as women academics do tend to carry more of the care burden in the home, their paid labour has been disproportionately interrupted by the pandemic. While publications are not the only form, nor necessarily the most important form of academic activity that has been impacted, the drop in women's publications is one clearly observable way in which existing inequities in academia have been amplified during the pandemic. Publication, along with grant, citation (Ghiasi et al., 2015) tenure (Antecol et al., 2018), pay and promotion (Huppatz et al., 2020) gender gaps predate the pandemic. These disparities are enabled by a number of organisational factors, including sexist academic cultures that overwhelming reward the individualistic, entrepreneurial, competitive, unencumbered worker, for whom excellence is associated with high quantities of outputs and funding, rather than quality, care and collegiality (O'Conner & O'Hagan, 2016; Huppatz et al., 2018). However, they have also overwhelmingly been associated with women academics' unpaid care obligations – with women taking on more care work within the home, and therefore having less time available for research (Misra et al., 2012). The pandemic, in removing the critical care infrastructures and support systems that academics, who are also primary carers, have in place in order to engage in paid employment, and in providing some unencumbered workers with further space and time to devote to research, has reminded us that these workplace and domestic norms still exist, and has exacerbated the gender inequities that both underpin and result from them.

Periera (2021) points out that the intensification of care labour for academics during the pandemic has not only occurred in the home, but also in the workplace: those who engage in pastoral care for staff and students have been overwhelmed with an extra care burden. The devastation of illness, death, isolation, financial hardship and overwork, caused by COVID-19, has led to an increase in stress and mental health issues for students and staff. In addition, the introduction of remote and online learning has demanded new ways of teaching, learning and communicating. Both of these developments have necessitated further collegial workplace practice and workplace care. Although we do not wish to conflate care with women, again, it is well documented that women tend to do this type of 'housekeeping' (Macfarlane and Burg, 2019) labour in higher education institutions, and so it follows that they have shouldered the majority of this work during the pandemic. Unfortunately, institutional housekeeping labour, while clearly vital to the wellbeing of the university community, constitutes what Babcock and co-authors (2017) describe as 'low promotability' work – it does not contribute to career advancement for those who carry out the pastoral care and actually detracts from academics' capacity to engage in 'high promotability' tasks such as research activities, which further explains the publication gap. While this type of care labour is essential to a collegial and ethical culture, when it comes to evaluating productivity and assessing for promotion, care labour is not sufficiently valued by universities (Huppatz et al., 2020). Universities, as with the broader capitalist system, are fundamentally flawed, in that they do not appreciate the care labour on which they depend. It has therefore been argued that the pandemic will have negative impacts on the career trajectories of women academics for some time to come (Minello, 2020), and that it is crucial that these impacts be tracked through research and ameliorated via institutional support (Myers et al., 2020), so that the COVID-19 shock is not left to individual academics to manage (Nash and Churchill, 2020).

Lessons learned: a research agenda for COVID-19 and society

The unusual situation under COVID lockdown revealed the contingent nature of women's employment and how, without adequate social and workplace supports and reliable care infrastructure, it takes second place behind the employment of male partners. It starkly underlined how necessary external care services are to families, and also that schools are part of a 'critical infrastructure of care' (Collins et al., 2021, p. 1), without which women's capacity to participate in employment is severely hindered.

Reduced working hours and unemployment will further impact women's economic security, possibly 'for decades to come' (Sasser Modestino, 2020), especially in contexts where significant gender pay gaps already existed, and where women were more likely to experience employment precarity, underemployment, unemployment, financial distress and poverty. Sasser Modestino (2020) warns that the lack of childcare and women's corresponding employment decisions may even set gender equity back a generation.

The long-term economic and social costs of the pandemic for women must therefore be monitored and mitigated, and a robust care crisis research agenda must continue. Following on from our case studies, we would like to make a series of recommendations for a research agenda for COVID-19 and society, that relate to our two areas of focus – domestic labour and the academy.

Recommendation one: reimagine the interconnections between domestic labour, the economy, social policies and workplace practices

Research into women in the labour force must be complemented by research that quantifies and monitors domestic labour in the home. A major reason housework and care is 'invisible' to policy makers and employers is that it is not regularly counted. We need up-to-date and reliable information about the time that it takes, and who is doing it. This would allow research to quantify both the combined burden of paid work and unpaid domestic work and care, and the trade-offs women and families make between the two forms of labour. At the macro-level, it would mean researchers could measure, calculate and analyse the trade-offs governments make between women's economic participation and having to provide more publicly funded care services. The best source of information on this is nationally representative time use surveys, which use time diaries to capture information about everything people do over the course of the day (Gershuny and Sullivan, 1998). Direct information from within households is needed to counteract the dominant tendency to view gender equality through the lens of employment, which obscures the value of care and reinforces the idea that only paid work is productive and effortful labour (Suh and Folbre, 2017).

Empirical research tracking domestic labour through the pandemic recovery would help keep gendered divisions of care on the policy agenda and provide important robust new evidence for decision making. Crises can challenge prior thinking and allow new ideas to emerge (van Barneveld et al., 2020). The neoliberal approach that underpinned the pre-existing care deficit (Ehrenreich and Hochschild, 2002; Livnat and Braslavsky, 2020) was challenged and stress tested during the pandemic. As the health crisis unfolded, the Australian government was temporarily willing to make childcare free to parents, subsidise aged care homes to help retain workers and give allowances to families who took elders out of facilities to be cared for at home (Craig and Churchill, 2020). This was implicit recognition that care work is a vital social and economic good whether it is paid or unpaid (Folbre, 2012), and that rather than being a private matter for families, care is essential, productive and a collective social concern (Fraser and Jaeggi, 2018). The interventions were quite a departure from standard policy, and the changes were only temporary. To engender longer lasting and more ambitious change requires robust research and evidence-based advocacy on how to reset the balance of paid work and the work of unpaid domestic labour and care. As part of this, we need international comparative research, so connections can be drawn between socio-political and employment context and help identify best practice across differing policy responses.

Making visible the time and effort involved in domestic labour and care, and situating it within policy context, is important to avoid creating perverse outcomes for women, families and the economy. For example, Australian state and federal governments spend AUD$90 billion a year on education and training yet there is mass underutilisation of women's education (ABS, 2019); Australian tax and childcare policies encourage women's part time work, because when day-care costs for more than three days a week are factored in, most mothers incur effective marginal tax rates near 100 per cent of their income (Wood et al., 2020); largely due to this part time work, more older women now live in poverty despite aged pension and superannuation subsidies costing the government over $45 billion annually (AHRC, 2019). The COVID-19 recovery is an opportunity to re-evaluate the counterproductive policies hampering women's economic opportunity and security and replace them with measures that acknowledge the social value of care.

Another research focus should be how the increasingly unpredictable and precarious labour market affects the domestic. There is a large and growing body of research and commentary on the 'future of work', including the implications of globalisation, technological change and the digital economy for underemployment and precarious work (Kalleberg, 2018), but little recognition that the shadow of labour market change is the future of family, care and social reproduction. Established economic assumptions and policy principles have proven flawed, undermining the idea that market competition and economic growth will promote wellbeing for all (Stiglitz et al., 2019). Women are disproportionately in occupational sectors with low-paid and insecure work, and with more people in the gig economy, doing casual work, piece work or on temporary contracts, we need to better understand the impacts of multiple job holding, underemployment, split shifts and multiple work sites (Churchill and Craig, 2019; Preston and Wright, 2020). With the unsustainable contradictions and gender blindness of the neoliberal era increasingly apparent following COVID-19, research on the domestic implications of the disrupting labour market is vital to understand the implications for the future of care.

Recommendation two: reimagine academia through recovery

Returning now to the narrower focus on the academy, researchers must continue to gather data on the ways in which the pandemic has exacerbated existing workforce inequalities, and the long-term consequences of the pandemic will need to be ascertained. While many universities have already taken steps to soften the impact of COVID-19 on researcher activity, and government grant schemes have extended timeframes (Myers et al., 2020), more could be done. Once again, in devising methods to mitigate the effects of the pandemic, there is an opportunity for us to reconsider existing policy and practice. Researchers and universities must address the plight of carers in ways that do not conflate women with motherhood (Periera, 2021) or reproduce heteronorms; however, they should understand how gender and care intersect. Both researchers and institutions might consider how workplaces could continue to provide more flexible work arrangements for staff with care responsibilities, offer affordable childcare and eldercare to workers and to better consider care interruptions in research workloads and performance assessments. This is not a time to be reducing existing gender equity and diversity measures, nor to cut childcare services, as some institutions have done in a bid to halt financial losses (Nash and Churchill, 2020).

When responding to the pandemic, universities must not adopt policy and practice that unwittingly set back women's gains in terms of career progression, tenure and pay within the academy. Crucially, many feminist academics have pointed to how competitive, neoliberal academic work cultures, which prioritise speedy, quantitative indicators of 'excellence', are particularly unfriendly to those workers who do not align with the white, heterosexual, middle-class, able bodied masculine ideal (O'Conner and O'Hagan, 2016; Huppatz et al., 2018). Therefore, any response to the pandemic should look to solutions that do not further normalise and celebrate these problematic values and norms of academic capitalism. For example, Periera (2021) points to how responses to interruptions in the careers of academics must avoid reifying publications as the only or most important aspect of academic labour that has been impacted.

Such a response should itself be informed by an ethics of care, in that collective wellbeing, rather than individual competition, is prioritised in research, teaching and leadership practice (Corbera et al., 2020). This is an opportunity to acknowledge care labour in all its forms – outside of the academy but also within the academy. This is a moment at which universities might revaluate how they reward teaching, mentoring and other service work, which currently count for little in terms of promotion (Misra et al., 2012), but are pertinent to an ethical, equitable and thriving university, especially when recovering from the pandemic. Thus, this is a time to reconsider how feminised academic care labour is valued within the academy, alongside research activities.

In suggesting a research agenda for the study of gender in academia, we are addressing both institutions and higher education researchers. Laube (2021) suggests that universities should listen to feminist sociologists in understanding the challenges that the pandemic has posed as well as seeking solutions, as these 'experts within their own ranks' are best placed to analyse organisational culture and avoid reproducing old mistakes. This is a pivotal moment for higher education scholars to take up engaged research in their own institutions and aid in the recovery process.

Recommendation three: reimagine the distribution of care through recovery

In addressing each of these case study areas, and looking beyond, we have an opportunity to apply an ethics of care to our research. Branicki (2020) argues that responses to the coronavirus pandemic, whether individual, organisational or policy based, should not just centre on the problem of care; the responses should themselves be informed by a feminist ethics of care. In relation to both case studies, we have suggested that there is an opportunity to address pre-existing inequities. Branicki (2020) suggests that Carol Gilligan's theory of the ethic of care provides the language from which crisis management could truly reconsider existing norms and institutional arrangements (for more on crisis management see Dittmer and Lorenz's chapter). Crisis management should move beyond containment and measurement, to 'provide a care-based concern for all crisis affected people' (Branicki, 2020, p. 872). This form of 'feminist crisis management might emphasize a relational logic grounded in preserving and extending relationships through a crisis through caring and seeing opportunities for a crisis to lead to transformation' (Branicki, 2020, p. 880). The COVID-19 care crisis is an opportunity to do gender and care differently; it is an opportunity to reformulate relationships, lessen the care burden and improve lives.

The consequences of ignoring or devaluing socially necessary unpaid work and care are substantial both for those who do this work and for societies as a whole (Folbre, 2012; Fraser and Jaeggi, 2018). For individuals, being disproportionately responsible for non-market work in a monetised economy that values little else has serious financial and psychological risks (Lewis, 2009), which can only be avoided if it is shared more equally, and if the social value of it is recognised (Folbre, 2012). Comprehensive work-family supports are needed as part of the basic social infrastructure to support the provision of socially necessary non-market work. Analysing workforce participation and unpaid social reproduction together would show the combined productive value of both, so debates about national productivity will be better informed. Too much work of either type can crowd out time for other important activities and apparent gains in national productivity may not only be illusory, but cause costly social depletion in wellbeing, health and social connectedness (Rai et al., 2014). If the future is to involve employment on equal terms for all genders, then the division of unpaid work and care also must be fair and sustainable (Goode's chapter in this book explicitly references the future). Furthermore, governments should share the costs of making it workable. Women cannot manage this on their own. Nor is it possible to leave this challenge to overstretched families. To map out a more sustainable future we need to redistribute the costs and demands of care not only more equally between men and women, but also more equally between families, employers and governments.

Concluding thoughts

The care crisis is expansive. There is evidence of a care deficit in our own homes and in our workplaces, academia being just one example. Here we have drawn upon two case studies – domestic labour and academia – to examine how the care crisis manifests in specific, gendered, ways and has been exacerbated by COVID-19. The coronavirus has brought our attention to, and deepened, serious gender inequalities: women are bearing the brunt of the unpaid care labour and this is having consequence for their capacity to participate in paid work and for their wellbeing. Both cases reveal the ways in which organisations and families reinforce the care deficit and rely on women to fill the care gap.

As we emerge from the COVID-19 crisis we must take stock of the damage but also take the opportunity to research and advocate in new ways and with more momentum. We have made some recommendations in this chapter on where we might start in terms of domestic labour: patterns in unpaid domestic labour must be recorded and made visible, counteracting an overemphasis on employment in government policy; work and care policies must be reassessed for their intended and unintended contributions to the care gap, and compared with their international counterparts; and the impact of precarious and changing labour markets upon domestic labour arrangements must be assessed. In terms of a research agenda for academia, we have suggested that researchers must continue to monitor the impacts of the coronavirus on the workforce, and point to ways in which the pandemic has worsened existing inequities; researchers must be advocates in their own universities, and ensure that any institutional responses do not reproduce damaging workplace norms; and in turn, universities are in a unique position in that they have expert data collectors, analysts and theorists in their own ranks, and so they should look to their own researchers in strategising for recovery. For both case studies, we have suggested that examining and re-examining existing structures and cultures, and offering structural and cultural solutions, is essential. We have suggested that a feminist ethics of care should be applied in the very manner in which we approach this research, and we have proposed that a comprehensive research agenda would look to how work-family support structures should be made part of our basic social infrastructure, supported by governments, workplaces and economies.

Our analysis and discussion here have pertained to two very specific areas of scholarship, and we have not spoken in any detail about the raced and classed dimensions to this care crisis, or the widening inequities in the global flow of care work. Nor have we discussed the poor working conditions and pay in our critical care infrastructure workforce – in our childcare, schools, hospitals and aged care facilities – all of which are important dimensions to the care deficit. In short, this social problem is so extensive that it is beyond the scope of one book chapter. This makes the need for new research all the more pressing.

References

ABS (Australian Bureau of Statistics). (2019). Population. *https://www.abs.gov.au/Population*.

AHRC. (2019). *Older Women's Risk of Homelessness: Background Paper Exploring a Growing Problem*. Australian Human Rights Commission Report. ISBN: 978-1-925917-01-7.

AIHW. (2019). *Australia's Welfare Report 2019*. The Australian Institute of Health and Welfare: Canberra.

Altintas, E. & Sullivan, O. (2016). 50 Years of Change Updated: Cross-national Gender Convergence in Housework. *Demographic Research 35*(16), 455–70.

Andrew, A., Cattan, S., Costa Dias, M., Farquharson, C., & Kraftman, L. (2020). Inequalities in Children's Experiences of Home Learning During the COVID-19 Lockdown in England *Fiscal Studies 41*(3), 653–83.

Antecol, H., Bedard, K., & Stearns, J. (2018). Equal but Inequitable: Who Benefits from Gender-neutral Tenure Clock Stopping Policies? *The Economics Review 108*(9), 2420–41.

Babcock, L., Recalde, M., Vesterlund, L., & Wingart, L. (2017). Gender Differences in Accepting and Receiving Requests for Tasks with Low Promotability. *American Economic Review 107*(3), 714–47.

Branicki, L. (2020). COVID-19, Ethics of Care and Feminist Crisis Management. *Gender, Work and Organization 27*, 872–83.

Carlson, D.L., Petts, R., & Pepin, J. (2020). *US Couples' Divisions of Housework and Childcare During COVID-19 Pandemic*. SocArXiv. https://osf.io/preprints/socarxiv/jy8fn/

Churchill, B. & Craig, L. (2019). Gender in the Gig Economy: Men and Women Using Digital Platforms to Secure Work in Australia. *Journal of Sociology 55*(4), 741–61.

Collins, C., Ruppaner, L., Landivar, L., & Scarborough, W. (2021). The Gendered Consequences of a Weak Infrastructure of Care: School Reopening Plans and Parents' Employment During the COVID-19 Pandemic. *Gender & Society*, online first. https://journals-sagepub-com.ezproxy.uws.edu.au/doi/10.1177/08912432211001300

Corbera, E., Anguelovski, I., Honey-Rosés, J., & Ruiz-Mallén, I. (2020). Academia in the Time of COVID-19: Towards an Ethics of Care, *Planning Theory & Practice 21*(2), 191–9.

Craig, L. (2020). Coronavirus, Domestic Labour and Care: Gendered Roles Locked Down. *Journal of Sociology 56*(4), 684–92.

Craig, L. & Brown, J. (2017). Feeling Rushed: Gendered Time Quality, Work Hours, Work Schedules and Spousal Crossover. *Journal of Marriage and Family 79*(1), 225–42.

Craig, L., Brown, J., & Jun, J. (2020). Fatherhood, Motherhood and Time Pressure in Australia, Korea and Finland. *Social Politics: International Studies in Gender, State and Society 27*(2), 312–36.

Craig, L., Brown, J., Strazdins, L., & Jun, Y. (2020). Fatherhood, Motherhood and Time Pressure. *Social Politics 27*(2), 312–36.

Craig, L. & Churchill, B. (2020). Working and Caring at Home: Gender Differences in the Effects of Covid-19 on Paid and Unpaid Labor in Australia. *Feminist Economics 27*(1–2), 310–26.

Craig, L. & Churchill, B. (2021a). Dual-earner Parent Couples' Work and Care During COVID-19. *Gender, Work & Organization 28*(S1), 66–79.

Craig, L. & Churchill, B. (2021b). Unpaid Work and Care During COVID-19: Subjective Experiences of Same-Sex Couples and Single Mothers in Australia. *Gender & Society 35*(2), 233–43.

Craig, L., Ravn, S., & Churchill, B. (forthcoming). *Making Education Work for Women*. Report to the Melbourne Lord Mayor's Charitable Foundation.

Cui, R., Hao, D., & Feng, Z. (2020). *Gender Inequality in Research Productivity During the COVID-19 Pandemic*. SSRN, 1–30. https://papers.ssrn.com/sol3/papers.cfm?abstract_id=3623492

Doucet, A. (2020) Father Involvement, Care, and Breadwinning: Genealogies of Concepts and Revisioned Conceptual Narratives. *Genealogy 4*(1), 14.

Ehrenreich, B. & Hochschild, A. (2002). *Global Woman: Nannies, Maids and Sex Workers in the New Economy*. Metropolitan Books/Henry Holt and Company, 1–14.

Fazackerley, A. (2020). Women's Research Plummets During Lockdown – But Articles from Men Increase. *The Guardian*, 12 May. https://www.theguardian.com/education/2020/may/12/womens-research-plummets-during-lockdown-but-articles-from-men-increase

Feng, Z. & Savani, K. (2020). Covid-19 Created a Gender Gap in Perceived Work Productivity and Job Satisfaction: Implications for Dual-career Parents Working from Home. *Gender in Management 35*(7/8), 719–36.

Folbre, N. (2012). *For Love or Money: Care Provision in the United States*. Russell Sage Foundation.

Fraser, N. & Jaeggi, R. (2018). *Capitalism: A Conversation in Critical Theory*. Polity Press.

Gershuny, J. & Sullivan. O.O. (1998). The Sociological Uses of Time-use Diary Analysis. *European Sociological Review 14*(1), 69–85.

Ghiasi, G., Larivière, V., & Sugimoto, C.R. (2015). On the Compliance of Women Engineers with a Gendered Scientific System. *PLoS ONE 10*(12), 1–19.

Giurge, L.M., Whillans, A.V., & Yemiscigil, A. (2021). A Multi-country Perspective on Gender Differences in Time Use During COVID-19. *Proceedings of the National Academy of Sciences (PNAS) 118*(12). doi.org/10.1073/pnas.2018494118

HILDA (Household, Income and Labour Dynamics in Australia Survey). (2019). *The Household, Income and Labour Dynamics in Australia Survey: Selected Findings from Waves 1 to 17.* Melbourne Institute: Applied Economic & Social Research. https://melbourneinstitute.unimelb.edu.au/__data/assets/pdf_file/0011/3127664/HILDA-Statistical-Report-2019.pdf

Huppatz, K., Sang, K., & Napier, J. (2018). If You Put Pressure on Yourself Then That's Your Responsibility: Mother's Experience of Maternity Leave and Flexible Work in the Academy. *Gender, Work & Organization 26*(6), 772–88.

Huppatz, K., Townley, C., Bansel, P., & Denson, N. (2020). *Redressing the Promotion Gap.* Vice-Chancellor's Gender Equality Fund Final Report, Western Sydney University. https://www.westernsydney.edu.au/__data/assets/pdf_file/0008/1762874/Final_Report_Redressing_the_Promotion_Gap_16122019.pdf

Kalleberg, A. (2018). *Precarious Lives: Job Insecurity and Well-being in Rich Democracies.* Polity Press.

Laube, H. (2021). COVID-19 Makes Transforming the Academy More Urgent. *Gender & Society Blog,* 30 March. https://gendersociety.wordpress.com/2021/03/30/covid-19-makes-transforming-the-academy-more-urgent/

Lewis, J. (2009). *Work–family Balance, Gender and Policy.* Edward Elgar.

Livnat, I. & Braslavsky, P. (2020). Who Takes Care of 'Care?' *Gender, Work & Organization 27*(2), 270–7.

Macfarlane, B. & Burg, D. (2019). Women Professors and the Academic Housework Trap. *Journal of Higher Education Policy and Management 41*(3), 262–74.

Matthewman, S. & Huppatz, K. (2020). A Sociology of Covid-19. *Journal of Sociology 56*(4), 507–15.

Minello, A. (2020). The Pandemic and the Female Academic. *Nature Briefing,* 3 May. https://www.nature.com/articles/d41586-020-01135-9

Misra, J., Lundquist, J., & Templer, A. (2012). Gender, Work Time, and Care Responsibilities Among Faculty. *Sociological Forum 27*(2), 300–23.

Mooi-Reci, I. & Risman, B. (2021). The Gendered Impacts of Covid-19: Lessons and Reflections. *Gender & Society,* online first: https://journals-sagepub-com.ezproxy.uws.edu.au/doi/full/10.1177/08912432211001305

Myers, K., Tham, W.Y., Yin, Y., Cohodes, N., Thursby, J., Thursby, M., Schiffer, P., Walsh, J., Lakhani, K., & Wang, D. (2020). Unequal Effects of the COVID-19 Pandemic on Scientists. *Nature Human Behaviour 4,* 880–3, 15 July. https://www.nature.com/articles/s41562-020-0921-y

Nash, M. & Churchill, B. (2020). Caring During COVID-19: A Gendered Analysis of Australian University Responses to Managing Remote Working and Caring Responsibilities. *Gender, Work & Organization 27*(5), 833–46.

Nieuwenhuis, R. & Yerkes, M. (2021). Workers' Well-being in the Context of the First Year of the COVID-19 Pandemic. *Community, Work & Family 24*(2), 226–35.

O'Connor, P. & O'Hagan, C. (2016). Excellence in University Academic Staff Evaluation: A Problematic Reality? *Studies in Higher Education 41*(11), 1943–57.

Periera, M. M. (2021). Researching Gender Inequalities in Academic Labour During the COVID-19 Pandemic: Avoiding Common Problems and Asking Different Questions. *Gender, Work & Organization 28*(2), 498–509.

Perry-Jenkins, M. & Gerstel, N. (2020). Work and Family in the Second Decade of the 21st Century. *Journal of Marriage and the Family 82*(February), 420–53.

Petts, R., Carlson, D., & Pepin, J. (2020). A Gendered Pandemic: Childcare, Home Schooling, and Parents' Employment During COVID-19. *Gender, Work & Organization 28*(2), 515–34.

Power, K. (2020). The COVID-19 Pandemic Has Increased the Care Burden of Women and Families. *Sustainability: Science, Practice and Policy 16*(1), 67–73. DOI: 10.1080/15487733.2020.1776561

Preston, A. & Wright, R. (2020). Exploring the Gender Difference in Multiple Job Holding. *Southern Economic Journal 85*(4), 1217–42.

Rai, S.M., Hoskyns, C., & Thomas, D. (2014). Depletion: The Cost of Social Reproduction. *International Feminist Journal of Politics 16*, 297–317.

Salk, R., Hyde, J., & Abramson, L. (2017). Gender Differences in Depression in Representative National Samples: Meta-Analyses of Diagnoses and Symptoms. *Psychological Bulletin 143*(8), 783–822.

Sasser Modestino, A. (2020). Coronavirus Child-care Crisis Will Set Women Back a Generation. *The Washington Post*. 15 April 2021. https://www.washingtonpost.com/us-policy/2020/07/29/childcare-remote-learning-women-employment/

Schieman, S., Badawy, P.J., Milkie, M.A., & Bierman, A. (2021). Work-Life Conflict During the COVID-19 Pandemic. *Socius*. DOI: 10.1177/2378023120982856

Sevilla, A. & Smith, S. (2020). Baby Steps: The Gender Division of Childcare During the COVID-19 Pandemic. *IZA Discussion Paper 13302*, 1–29.

Skountridaki, L., Zschomler, D., Marks, A., & Mallett, O. (2020). Work-Life Balance for Home-Based Workers Amidst a Global Pandemic. *The Work-Life Balance Bulletin 4*(2), 16–22.

Stiglitz, J., Fitoussi J-P., & Durand, M. (2019). *Measuring What Counts*. U.S: The New Press.

Strazdins, L., Broom, D., Banwell, C., McDonald, T., & Skeat, H. (2011). Time limits? Reflecting and Responding to Time Barriers for Healthy, Active Living. *International Journal of Health Promotion, 26*(1), 46–54.

Suh, J. & Folbre, N. (2017). Time, Money, and Inequality. *Œconomia. History, Methodology, Philosophy 7*(1), 3–24.

van Barneveld, K., Quinlan, M., Kriesler, P., Junor, A., Baum, F., Chowdhury, A., Junankar, P.N., Clibborn, S., Flanagan, F., Wright, C.F., Friel, S., Halevi, J., & Rainnie, A. (2020). The COVID-19 Pandemic: Lessons on Building More Equal and Sustainable Societies. *Economic and Labour Relations Review 31*(2): 133–157. URL (consulted June 19, 2020): https://doi.org/10.1177/1035304620927107

Williams, J.C., Blair-Loy, M., & Berdahl, J. (2013). Cultural Schemas, Social Class, and the Flexibility Stigma. *Journal of Social Issues 69*(2), 209–34.

Wood, D., Griffiths, K., & Emslie, O. (2020). *Cheaper Childcare: A Practical Plan to Boost Female Workforce Participatio*. Grattan Institute Report No. 2020-11, Grattan Institute Melbourne.

World Health Organization. (2016). *Out of the Shadows: Making Mental Health a Global Development Priority*. http://www.who.int/mental_health/advocacy/wb_background_paper.pdf?ua=1 Retrieved November 26, 2016.

Xue, B. & McMunn, A. (2021). Gender Differences in Unpaid Care Work and Psychological Distress in the UK Covid-19 Lockdown. *PLOS One. 16*(3). doi.org/10.1371/journal.pone.0247959

10 The futures of qualitative research in the COVID-19 era: experimenting with creative and digital methods

Clare Southerton, Marianne Clark,
Ash Watson and Deborah Lupton

Introduction

As COVID-19 health and safety restrictions have disrupted face-to-face qualitative research methods, many researchers have been left seeking alternative ways to engage with their participants and their field sites. At the same time, qualitative research is well placed to respond to the nuanced ways this significant event has impacted daily life, using practices attuned to the specificities of different contexts and lived experiences. Using digital technologies such as video calling to conduct research remotely has been widely seen as a way to adapt existing research methods to respond to the risks of our new COVID-19 world. Beyond working on adapting traditional methods, there has also been an opportunity to experiment with innovative and creative methods during this period.

While these methods, for many, have been taken up out of necessity, this chapter makes a case for considering the opportunity offered to rethink the empirical grounds of qualitative research, even once the threat of a pandemic passes (and on the prospects of being 'post-pandemic' see Dittmer and Lorenz in this volume). We draw on three case studies to consider the capacities of creative and digital research methods: a digital photo-diary study exploring fitness practices during pandemic lockdown; a qualitative analysis of health information content and sharing practices on the social media app TikTok; and a project employing online creative writing workshops to elicit participants' feelings and practices concerning their personal data.

The analysis of our empirical research relies on 'thinking with theory' (Jackson and Mazzei, 2012). In our case, this involves using sociomaterial perspectives that draw principally on vital materialism scholarship espoused in non-western and Indigenous philosophies and feminist materialism. Non-western and Indigenous philosophies have traditionally recognised the distributed and relational nature of human embodiment, agency and subjectivity as part of their worldviews (Hernández et al., 2020; Rots, 2017; and see Lambert's chapter in this volume for discussion of Indigenous worldviews and research pertaining to Indigenous Peoples). Scholars contributing to feminist materialism perspectives,[1] including Donna Haraway (2016), Jane Bennett (2020), Rosi Braidotti (2019) and Karen Barad (2007), have more recently developed a comparable more-than-human approach that builds on the philosophy of Spinoza and Deleuze and Guattari.

Vital materialism, as explained in this scholarship, adopts a perspective that brings ontologies, epistemologies and ethical issues together as inextricable: as Barad (2007) puts it, it is an onto-ethico-epistemological position. Vital materialism views humans as always already more than human, entangled in relations and connections not only with other people but also non-human agents, including other animals, plants, places and non-organic things. In this conceptualisation, human–non-human assemblages are emergent and dynamic: constantly changing as people move through their everyday lives in both time and space. Vitalities and vibrancies such as affective forces and agencies are generated with and through these assemblages, opening or closing capacities for action and human flourishing. We argue that bringing together vital materialism with innovative methods provides an opportunity to surface the ways that digital objects, bodies and practices are always implicated in the formation of subjects (Lupton, 2019). Digitised experiences are often conceptualised as disembodied in popular culture and even academic writing. As Hine (2015) reminds us, however, digital spaces are always encountered and experienced in multisensory and fleshly ways.

In this chapter, we show how the pandemic turn to digital and creative qualitative methods is an opportunity to reflect on how the sensory, bodily and habitual dimensions of more-than-human worlds may be attended to in research. We first provide a brief review of recent social inquiry responding to the sociomaterialities of the COVID-19 crisis and the methodological challenges posed by social-distancing conditions. We then present our three case studies, providing detailed accounts of the different methods used and considering the benefits and drawbacks of each. Finally, we discuss how the tumultuous events and consequences of the COVID-19 crisis offer an opportunity for rethinking research methods beyond simply managing COVID-19-related risk (for further discussion of the opportunities provided by the pandemic see the chapter by Matthewman). We consider how creative and digital research methods can help social researchers to reflect critically on knowledge production.

COVID-19 and sociomateriality

Scholars drawing on vital materialism theory have begun to explore the conceptual onto-ethico-epistemological dimensions of the COVID-19 crisis, drawing attention to the intersections and intra-actions (Barad, 2007) of humans with places such as the home, hospitals, natural environments and leisure spaces, and with objects such as face masks (Braidotti, 2020; Fullagar and Pavlidis, 2021; Lupton et al., 2021; Smith et al., 2020). A growing body of empirical social research has also appeared in response to the COVID-19 crisis. Some of this research has incorporated creative methods to examine how people have responded to the crisis and how the sociomaterial conditions of everyday life have shifted. For example, Olimpia Mosteanu (2021) used photography to document and analyse the role of windows in the London lockdown in supporting residents' wellbeing during this period of social isolation. Thorpe et al. (2021) engaged in poetic inquiry to explore new ethical considerations and concerns around body movement, breath, space and contagion in relation to COVID-19 risk in the contexts of Aotearoa/ New Zealand and Australia. Ernesto Priego and Peter Wilkins (2020) created autoethnographic comics to reflect their experiences of the pandemic. Taking digital spaces as their field site, Crystal Abidin and Jing Zeng (2020) explored how an online Asian community created solidarity and support during COVID-19 when racist attacks and xenophobia towards people of East Asian appearance became intensified during the pandemic (Wyver's chapter is devoted to the pandemic/race nexus).

Other researchers have experimented with digital and online methods to breach the distance between themselves and their research participants. After having to suddenly shift their Sydney-based ethnographic home visits to virtual visits mediated by video-calling apps and smartphones, Watson et al. (2021) investigated how their participants enacted intimacy and sociality via distance during the national lockdown by using the same technologies. Another digital method employed during COVID-19 restriction periods was that of zine-making workshops held online by Pollitt et al. (forthcoming). Using Zoom video conferencing to connect each participant working with materials such as paper, pens and glue at home, they led participants across diverse locations in creating zines in response to prompts about women's experiences of academic work during the crisis.

Inspired by this scholarship as we navigated the practicalities of maintaining our own research programs during COVID-19 conditions, we were prompted to re-design and reimagine a series of methods that accommodated the rapidly shifting research context. Embracing the potential of creative and digital methods, we thought carefully about what was available to us methodologically as we sought to answer a range of overarching research questions. Here, we share examples of these methods to illustrate the potential of thinking outside of the comfort zone and working at the intersections of theory and method.

Case studies

Digital photo diaries: exploring fitness practices during lockdown

Our first example focuses on an experimental digital photo diary method developed by Marianne Clark to explore people's movement practices during lockdown. The project was prompted by her personal observations in the eastern suburbs of Sydney. At the height of lockdown conditions in Australia's first wave of COVID-19 (April 2020), she noticed people engaging in outdoor spaces in new ways. Usually tranquil neighbourhoods were suddenly bustling with walkers and runners, and people could be seen working out in driveways and garages repurposed as impromptu gyms. At this time, exercise was one of the few allowable reasons for people to leave the house. Yet many beaches, fitness centres, organised sports and outdoor gyms were closed to limit the spread of the virus. These closures presented constraints to people seeking to achieve regular physical activity during the pandemic. Nevertheless, public health messaging encouraged people to remain active (World Health Organization, 2020a). These messages highlighted the importance of regular physical activity for supporting both mental and physical health in stressful conditions and provided general advice targeting individual behaviour. However, physical activity is always complex behaviour shaped by myriad social, economic, and material factors (Silk and Andrews, 2011). Pandemic physical activity messaging seemed to overlook these complexities, and Clark was curious as to how people negotiated different obstacles to create new exercise practices.

Given the centrality of the human body and its sensory and affective capacities in response to living in and through a health crisis, Clark was particularly inspired by sociomaterial frameworks that acknowledge the generativity of the material and more-than-human entities. Specifically, she was curious about how people engaged with indoor and outdoor spaces, digital technologies, and everyday objects to create new fitness routines in the sociomaterial context of the pandemic. This study was designed to explore how these heterogeneous forces were creatively re/assembled to produce movement practices and to surface the meanings these embodied practices held for people living in stressful times. With face-to-face research methods off the table, a methodological approach that accommodated the constraints of the pandemic was required. Clark also sought a method that could access the affective and embodied experiences afforded by movement not always easily articulated through language and text. At the same time, while pandemic conditions meant people's comfort and familiarity with a variety of digital platforms had increased, she was also mindful of the widespread experience of screen fatigue and wished to limit the demand on participants to spend more time in front of a screen.

Given these parameters, Clark developed an innovative digital photo diary method. This approach draws inspiration from visual methodologies such as photovoice (Wang and Burris, 1997) and photo elicitation (Harper, 2002) as well as written and audio diary methods often used in ethnographic research. Many of these methods come from sociological and anthropological traditions and are intended to generate rich research materials that capture insights into the everyday worlds of participants (Glaw et al., 2017; and see Wynn and Trnka's contribution for an extended discussion of this). Such methods also seek to privilege participants' perspectives and voices, allowing them to decide what is meaningful and to purposefully curate images and stories they deem important.

Elaborating on these methods, the digital photo diaries asked participants to take photos capturing moments that were somehow associated with their daily movement practices. No parameters on who or what was to appear in the photos were provided. Instead, this method sought to privilege participant perspective. Participants were also asked to share a brief story about the image, describe its meaning to them and articulate how it related to their movement experience. The diaries sought to alleviate the emphasis on text and language as a means to express and represent experience and also to capture meaningful moments across time and space that might otherwise be missed in an interview setting.

For the study, participants were recruited via social media outlets (for example, Facebook and Twitter). To be eligible, participants were required to be between 18 and 64 years of age, living in Australia and currently participating in at least

20 minutes of physical activity two or more times per week. Participants were also asked to confirm access to the technologies necessary to access email and to take and upload photographs.

The first stage of the project involved online interviews conducted over Zoom that also included a virtual tour of the physical activity space used. A total of 19 people participated in this portion of the study, ranging in age from 29 to 56 years. Participants included 12 women and 7 men. Ten people lived in Sydney, eight in Melbourne, Australia's two largest cities, and one in Newcastle, a mid-sized city north of Sydney. All participants were also invited to participate in the digital photo diaries. Eight people agreed: five women and three men. For this part of the project, participants were emailed daily for 7–10 days and required to submit a total of five entries. Each email contained a link to a Qualtrics form that asked participants to upload a digital photo inspired by or related to their physical activity experience that day. The connection between the photograph and physical activity was purposely broad and left to participants to interpret. Examples and prompts provided included:

(1) A piece of equipment, object or technology that plays a role in your movement practice
(2) A view or image that inspires or touches you while participating in your movement practice
(3) Any other people, animals, or settings that are meaningful to your movement practice in some way

Participants were then asked to provide information about the photograph, including:

(1) When and where the photo was taken
(2) Who and what appears in the photo
(3) Any other information they believe to be important

Finally, participants were invited to write a short narrative about what the photo means to them and why they were inspired to take it. Participants were asked to write at least one paragraph of text in the allotted space.

Everyone completed the five entries within 10 days for a total of 35 entries. Qualtrics forms were filled out completely, with no technological difficulties reported. An array of images emerged, ranging from photographs of fitness equipment such as running shoes and wetsuits, to indoor and outdoor spaces and natural and urban landscapes. As Figure 10.1 shows, these images captured both mundane settings (for example, lounge rooms, gardens, urban

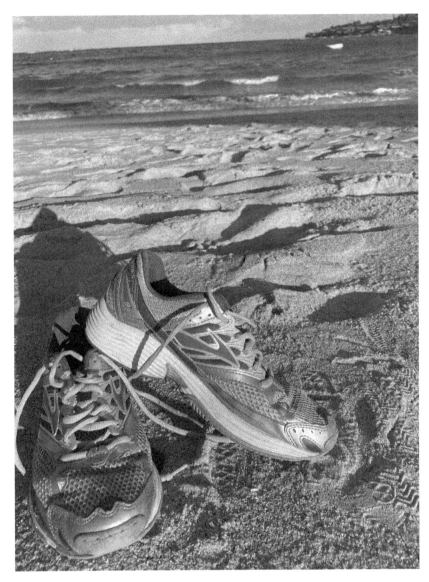

Figure 10.1   A photograph taken by a participant illustrating the importance of outdoor spaces and everyday fitness equipment like running shoes during the pandemic

sidewalks) and aesthetic landscapes (for example, coastlines, walking trails, green spaces).

To analyse the diaries, Clark oriented herself to the 'more-than-human' forces emerging in the photos and accompanying text. Stories and images pointed to the ways that every day practices and fitness-oriented movement practices are always entangled with histories, presents and futures and how they shift across time and space; what Barad (2007) refers to as 'spacetimemattering'. For example, participants noted how their personal histories and preferences for movement shaped their current practices as they sought to cope with the complex conditions of the pandemic and exist with uncertain futures. Stories surfaced of the entangled relations between humans and the more than human that are productive of everyday experiences and meanings. For example, domestic spaces such as lounge rooms and familiar fitness equipment such as rubber TheraBands and yoga mats came to matter in specific ways as they enabled daily movement practices that provided physical and emotional relief and release to participants. Additionally, movement for these participants was not about achieving an arbitrary health metric (for example, lowering blood pressure) or bodily aesthetic. Rather, improvised fitness routines emerged in response to the shifting and often stressful social, emotional and material conditions of daily life during the pandemic. Movement came to matter in new ways and far from being a utilitarian practice undertaken to preserve 'good health', it was imagined and experienced as a capacious practice that shifted the embodied way of being in the world during COVID-19. Therefore, this creative, digital visual method allowed Clark to capture the embodied, affective experiences of living through the pandemic, and to surface the ways these experiences emerge through the relations between more-than-human forces such as space, technology, objects and movement.

The use of digital photo diaries was meant to provide means of expression that complement or even exceed conventional logocentric approaches. However, these methods still rely on access to digital technologies and data, which is not always equitable. Research on digital inclusion in Australia has found that lower income, lower levels of education and living in a regional area can all reduce the likelihood of internet access. Aboriginal people, people with disabilities, older people and culturally and linguistically diverse migrants are also more likely to lack access to the internet (Thomas et al., 2020). Additionally, the design specificities of the Qualtrics platform meant the digital photo diary template was quite static, leaving little room for participants to decide how to share and represent their images and voice. Further consideration to questions of voice (Jackson and Mazzei, 2012) and experimentation with alternative platforms may further enrich this method.

Qualitative social media analysis: studying COVID-19 health information on TikTok

Our second case study is a digital ethnography conducted by Clare Southerton to examine the circulation of health information content on the social media app TikTok. TikTok is a short-form video-sharing app that saw a rapid rise in popularity in 2020 as many countries around the world were entering COVID-19 lockdowns (Chan, 2020). The platform's content is highly trend driven and often oriented around meme making, especially audio memes: that is, using the same sounds or music others have used to make referential content (Abidin, 2021).

As the COVID-19 pandemic unfolded, there was significant concern about the role of social media apps like TikTok in spreading misinformation about the coronavirus. The World Health Organization (2020b, p. 2) warned that populations around the globe were facing an 'infodemic': defined as 'an over-abundance of information – some accurate and some not – that makes it hard for people to find trustworthy sources and reliable guidance when they need it'. While there is an emerging scholarship exploring the potential of TikTok as a platform for disseminating health information (Comp et al., 2020; Eghtesadi and Florea, 2020), there has been little examination of how health information is shared on TikTok, especially by health professionals who use the app. Given that information is experienced not only cognitively but also affectively, Southerton also sought to develop a method for examining and becoming attuned to the ways engaging with these platforms involves practices that are bodily and multisensory.

To explore these practices and communities, Southerton conducted a digital ethnography on TikTok over several months in 2020. Digital ethnography adapts ethnographic methods to increasingly digital worlds, taking digital spaces such as social media platforms as field sites (Pink et al., 2015). Following Christine Hine's work on virtual ethnography, Southerton also drew on autoethnography as part of her practice, using her sensory experience of browsing the platform and watching TikToks 'as a source of insight into the unresolvable uncertainties and tensions that can be a part of the Internet experience' (Hine, 2015, p. 82). This method was chosen to develop a deeper understanding of how health information circulates on the app, by becoming attuned to the specificities of TikTok's dynamic environment. By being embedded in platform cultures, Southerton was able to develop what Anderson and Ash (2015, p. 46) describe as a 'qualitative vocabulary of thresholds and tipping points'.

Southerton undertook sessions of browsing the app, which usually lasted between one and three hours. Initially, she used the app's search function for keywords such as 'covid', 'coronavirus', 'doctor', 'nurse', 'healthcare worker'. After viewing videos (TikToks) found using these keywords, further content was identified by clicking on hashtags on these TikToks. Southerton also periodically read the comments on TikToks to gain a better understanding of the interactions between the creator and their audience. Fieldnotes were taken in the form of screenshots from the app and written notes reflecting on experiences on the app. Videos were also downloaded from TikTok to keep for later review.

TikTok customises content for its users based on a range of information collected by the app (TikTok, 2020). TikTok's personalisation and search algorithms are proprietary, and so it is not possible to access specific information about their workings. It is important to acknowledge, then, that content visible to Southerton on TikTok will have been shaped by this data collection, as well as the app settings, including language and the location of her smartphone in Australia, among other things. Furthermore, it is important to contextualise TikTok as a social space within broader issues of inequality of access that will shape the kinds of content on the app. As outlined earlier, access to the internet and digital technologies is lower among already marginalised groups, exacerbated existing economic, social and racial inequalities. However, digital inclusion remains high among young people (Thomas et al., 2020), and as such there remains considerable optimism among health professionals about TikTok's potential to reach young people (Comp et al., 2020).

There are a number of ethical issues to consider when analysing social media content. In this case, although the content is posted publicly, it remains important to consider what the intention of the content creator may have been with regards to visibility and what the risks could be for the creator and their work (Patterson, 2018). Despite the orientation of the platform towards virality and gaining attention, not all videos posted to the site are posted with large audiences in mind. Highfield and Leaver (2016) identify the risks of analysing visual content, cautioning that creators may unintentionally reveal personal information in their content and, therefore, researchers must evaluate content carefully. Anonymity, however, is not always the best strategy as some creators may prefer attribution for their creation. In this instance, Southerton elected not to identify specific videos or creators in findings, with the exception of high-profile creators who had reached a level of micro-celebrity such that it was safe to assume their videos were intended to reach a broad audience. However, she also was cautious not to describe any video in detail in research findings that did contain personal information about the creator. For example, if a video featured detailed information about where a creator lived or about their family, this information may not be appropriate to describe.

In analysing TikToks, Southerton employed a method that involved being attuned to the expressive qualities of the TikTok videos – watching some on repeat a number of times, as certain TikToks (especially those that are very short) would likely be viewed this way by users. This approach was oriented towards becoming attuned to the shifting affects throughout the video as it looped, with emergent elements of the video being notable on rewatching. This is an important aspect of the method, as on the app itself videos are played on continual repeat unless the users act to switch to the next video.

Using this method, Southerton was able to observe the ways that TikToks can be used to create the conditions for shared intimacy between creator and audience in the context of the pandemic. There were many qualities of the videos that showed a significant departure from existing communication strategies used by health professionals, even on social media. The content examined on TikTok explored the tensions, anxieties, discomfort and heightened emotions of the pandemic, with medical professionals filming videos immediately after significant events such as a death or offering intensely personal reflections on the impact of the pandemic on their work and everyday life. Many TikToks took the viewer into hospitals and other workplaces for medical professionals, giving behind-the-scenes glimpses of the clutter of medical machinery, instruments and other devices that make up these spaces. Other TikToks called attention to the way the virus is felt as a material thing, through videos that highlighted our new awareness of viral contagion and references to spit and other bodily fluids.

Certainly, this digital ethnographic approach has limitations in terms of what the research materials collected using this method can surface. Researchers using digital ethnographies are well placed to examine affordances, attention economies and felt experience of platforms – from an autoethnographic perspective – as well as the communities that emerge on and through them. However, this method is limited in what it can reveal about the motivations and experiences of users, as it relies on the insights the ethnographers themselves can glean from content and interactions. As such, in some cases, it may be appropriate to investigate a research question further with interviews with research participants, for example, to access these perspectives.

Creative writing workshops: examining participants' data feelings and practices

Our third case study comes from the 'Living with Personal Data' project, a sociological exploration of what people understand, feel and do with their personal digital data. Deborah Lupton, Mike Michael and Ash Watson comprised the research team. The project as originally designed involved home-based video ethnographies with 30 Sydney-based participants, and eight creative methods workshops with groups of 6 to 8 participants. Fieldwork ran from early 2020 to early 2021, beginning at a time in which the research team was faced with suddenly changing the in-progress and planned research methods so as to be able to continue the study when COVID-19 lockdowns were instituted (in Australia, the national lockdown began from March 2020). We re-designed our methods so that rather than taking place in person, as we had begun to do in the project, all activities were conducted online.

In what follows we take an example from the series of creative workshops, led by Watson, and the materials it generated as our focus. Our workshops centred the notion of 'data sense' (Lupton, 2019), meaning the combination of human senses, embodied feelings, digital sensors and social sense-making practices which shape and make personal data. After re-designing our methods and shifting to an online format, we facilitated workshops via the digital platform Zoom. While this change meant that participants could not be in a room together and easily see the creative artefacts that each of them generated in response to our prompts, there were several other advantages to going online instead. Organising the workshops became much easier, as we were not limited to a physical location that suited everyone. Further, we could bring together participants who lived in geographically disparate areas and, therefore, diverse social contexts: including people living in rural and remote Australia, who are often left out of social research because of their less accessible location. We did not completely relinquish 'hands-on' methods, however. We structured the online workshops around two 'analogue' activities; participants joined via their computers or mobile devices and had pens and paper with which they could write and draw in response to our prompts. By engaging participants in hands-on activities, we involved their bodies in more-than-digital ways (that is, with more than verbal discussion and 'beyond' their technological devices). These activities were also creative, and as such, engaged participants' senses as they imagined, made visible (through illustration), and wrote detailed stories about data and technologies.

Following introductions, each workshop began with a brainstorming activity: participants were given one minute to write down how they understand and define 'data' and 'personal data', followed by 15 to 20 minutes to collectively

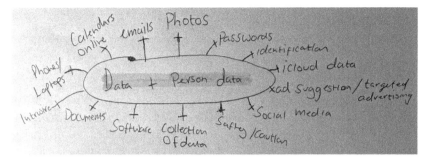

Figure 10.2   A mind-map drawn by a participant about 'data' and
                   'personal data'

discuss. This structure allowed discussion to build from immediately shared
perceptions of what data are and how data are made, as Figure 10.2 shows.

The findings from this initial activity showed how participants understood
personal data. Broadly, these understandings fell into three groupings.
Participants discussed *categorisations* of personal data (for example, personal,
identifiable, private and public), *types* of data (for example, information about
their finances, where they travel and live, whom they speak to or interact with
online, what they read or watch and what they buy) and *collections* of data
(for example, using terms such as observations, statistics, records, trends and
profiles). Groups also discussed how personal data were generated in their
everyday lives in active and passive ways, for example, through using emails,
step counters, social media, search engines, streaming services and maps as
well as via accessing buildings, taking public transport and moving through
public spaces embedded with cameras or sensors. Structuring the workshop
in this way thus had empirical and methodological value. The brainstorming
discussion worked to connect participants' understandings of personal data –
which can be abstracted – to their own everyday technology use, routines and
practices. Through this first activity, before the more creative second task,
personal data 'became' something material and situated for the group.

The second activity was unique in each workshop: verbally and via the Zoom
chat function, participants were given a creative prompt we had devised
about digital technologies and personal data, to which they had 10 minutes to
respond. One of these prompts was the following:

> Imagine a near future where facial recognition technology is everywhere; write
> about what these smart things and spaces are, and the impact this would have on

your life'. Imagine a near future in which smart objects and smart environments constantly scan your face using facial recognition software. What are these smart things? How would this technology make your life easier? Make your life harder?

Watson asked each group to discuss what they had created and their experiences of doing the activity until the end of the workshop time. As with the first activity, rather than leading with predetermined questions, Watson encouraged group discussion, asking participants to respond to others' creations, ideas, experiences, and perceptions and ask their own questions of others. Some participants directly shared what they had created by reading aloud and/ or by holding up their creations to their cameras, while others talked about what they had written or drawn and why.

The group discussion after this started with a discussion of *Black Mirror*, the speculative technology television series, and noted other similar dystopian texts including *Minority Report* and spy movies in general. These examples from mainstream popular culture shaped people's imaginaries of how a near-future world might feel. As they shared their responses to the prompts and discussed the thoughts these responses provoked, the group agreed 'literally anything' could become embedded with facial recognition technology. They focused more on how and why these technologies would be used: including for denying people access to public places, which Alex likened to a bouncer at a nightclub. Several participants also immediately extended from facial recognition devices themselves to what the outcomes of those devices would be, including public targeted advertising and the associated risks of other people seeing the potentially private interests/activities that were advertised. Alex posed the question to the group of rights to anonymity and privacy and how these may be flouted by facial recognition technology. Maddie added to this by saying in her written response to the prompt she had noted the impact that facial recognition could have on people 'trying to escape' from bad situations, and that personal hacking and tracking would be much easier if these technologies were more widely available to the public.

However, participants were just as ready to acknowledge the convenience and feelings of safety and reassurance offered by facial recognition technology. For example, according to one person's written response to the prompt:

> I think that facial recognition being everywhere will actually make Australia/the world a lot safer. In terms of crimes, hiring staff, going to major events, using services. People would be more self-conscious of the decisions that they make, and how they effect [sic] others . . . Will make life easier for a lot of people, as in say, for example, using ATM [automated teller machine] or paying for things. Can also help make life easier for people with disabilities; make daily life easier for them.

The group also discussed the impacts on people's practices if they knew such devices were ubiquitous and continually recording people's faces and movements while able to identify them instantaneously. They made reference to the recent US Capitol riots in Washington and how the increased use of facial recognition could potentially make a positive impact on crime in general. Courtney, who lives in the state of Victoria and lived through a second extended COVID-19 lockdown in 2020, added that facial recognition technology could potentially contribute to improved contract tracing processes by facilitating the easy identification of individuals. Watson probed the group about the feelings and emotions they expressed in their written responses to the prompts. It was notable that how people felt about the technology was strongly related to their perceptions of risk. Daniel, for instance, said he feels that your face is quite safe and not easily stolen or replicated, even with the use of facial recognition technologies, whereas Alex felt it was highly risky.

By analysing our findings using the vital materialist theories and approach detailed above, we were able to surface the constitutive entanglement of our participants' personal digital data with their domestic environments, routine practices, familial and social relationships and their future-oriented imaginaries. The findings from these activities showed what personal data *do* in our participants' lives, including what kinds of feelings, practices and relational dynamics data helps produce. Our findings also included what our participants imagine, feel, expect, resist, refuse, endure and enjoy about personal data and its generative processes. They gave us important insight into why participants care about personal data in the ways that they do and illuminated how data comes to matter in people's everyday lives.

Discussion and conclusion

Just as COVID-19 has unsettled everyday life and disrupted assumptions about the world and our relations to it, it has also unsettled our research and thinking practices, prompting us to imagine new ways of knowing and being. However, knowledge is always unsettled, emergent and uncertain (Barad, 2007) and the extraordinary conditions of COVID-19 have explicitly brought this into view. Adapting and re-designing our research methods in response to the COVID-19 crisis prompted us to grapple with the emergent and situated nature of inquiry and to examine our own understandings of how knowledge is produced, how research materials are generated and what types are meaningful for social inquiry.

As many scholars turn to creative and digital methods, it is important to acknowledge the rich history of these methods and their use in existing scholarship. As our case studies have illustrated, existing digital methods such as digital ethnography require the development of new skillsets for new 'field sites'. For example, Clark's case study developed the digital photo diary method by drawing on existing photovoice and photo elicitation methods, while the 'Living with Personal Data' project developed novel creative prompts that built on a longstanding literature about arts- and design-based methods for social inquiry. Importantly, our methods are deeply informed and inextricable from the theoretical approaches we engage. They are 'research creations' that involve assemblages of people with concepts, ideas, materials, place and space (Lupton and Watson, 2020). These frameworks emphasise the importance of 'response-ability', a concept elaborated by Haraway (2016) and Barad (2007) that refers to the capacity to respond thoughtfully to the conditions one encounters; the ability to respond to 'what matters' (Barad, 2007, p. 38). Haraway (2016, p. 34) describes response-ability as a practice, a careful 'cultivating collective knowing and doing'.

The methods we present here, although eclectic in approach, embody this orientation to response-ability. Our ability to respond emerges as a relational capacity – with our research topics, the digital, technological, affective and embodied, human, and more than human. The conditions of COVID-19 have prompted a rethinking of 'what matters', and so too has the need to think creatively about our methods during this time. As Christia and Chappell Lawson (2020) argue, among the challenges the pandemic has brought to the research community, there are also opportunities for innovation and adaptation. COVID-19 has prompted us to cultivate responsiveness as part of research practice beyond a crisis – to be equipped theoretically, methodologically and ethically to respond to multiple and shifting conditions that shape social life as the norm rather than as a risk to be managed. The creative and digital methods in our case studies call attention to the ways humans are always constituted within and through our environments. These methods, which creatively use digital tools to overcome physical distance, are always more than digital. We see the research encounter as constituted by sensing bodies, objects and relations, rather than only as individuated subjects who are mediated by technologies. Our case studies have highlighted the ways that creative and digital methods can be taken up to consider how the COVID-19 pandemic is felt, integrated into practices and embodied, as well as thought and discursively understood.

While COVID-19 conditions prompted a pragmatic reimagining of research, we argue this also prompts a deeper rethinking of how we understand knowledge production and its entangled sociomaterial and political processes. No longer able to turn to familiar methodological toolboxes, researchers are called upon to identify and create 'new' ways to engage in processes of knowing, being and doing. In our experiences, creative digital and arts-based methods enabled our research projects to continue and moved us to rethink the ontological and epistemological underpinnings of our inquiry. This is particularly important for those researchers engaging with sociomaterialist approaches, as such perspectives prompt an unsettling of the conventional ways in which we 'do' research (Lupton and Watson, 2020; St. Pierre et al., 2016; Thorpe et al., 2020). Such emergent approaches are not of course 'new'. Yet the uncertain and shifting conditions of the COVID-19 crisis underlined the continuously shifting and evolving nature of knowledge itself (not just in COVID-19 times): a fluidity, instability and dynamism that are not always assumed or acknowledged in research. In this time of uncertainty, we have an opportunity to think creatively not only about our methods but what it is we work with to examine them.

Note

1   The chapter in this book by Huppatz and Wynn analyses care through a feminist lens.

References

Abidin, C. (2021). Mapping Internet Celebrity on TikTok: Exploring Attention Economies and Visibility Labours. *Cultural Science Journal 12* (1), 77–103.

Abidin, C. & Zeng, J. (2020). Feeling Asian Together: Coping with #COVIDRacism on Subtle Asian Traits. *Social Media + Society*. https://doi.org/10.1177/2056305120948223.

Anderson, B. & Ash, J. (2015). Atmospheric Methods. In P. Vannini (Ed.) *Non-Representational Methodologies* (pp. 44–61). Routledge.

Barad, K. (2007). *Meeting the Universe Halfway: Quantum Physics and the Entanglement of Matter and Meaning.* Duke University Press.

Bennett, J. (2020). *Influx and Efflux: Writing Up with Walt Whitman.* Duke University Press.

Braidotti, R. (2019). *Posthuman Knowledge.* Polity.

Braidotti, R. (2020). 'We' Are in This Together, but We Are Not One and the Same. *Journal of Bioethical Inquiry 17*, 465–9.

Chan, J. (2020). Top Apps Worldwide for April 2020 by Downloads. *Sensor Tower.* https://sensortower.com/blog/top-apps-worldwide-april-2020-by-downloads.

Christia, F. & Lawson, J. C. (2020). Training the COVID-19 Cohort: Adapting and Preserving Social Science Research. *Items: Insights from the Social Sciences.* 30 July.

https://items.ssrc.org/covid-19-and-the-social-sciences/social-research-and-insecurity/training-the-covid-19-cohort-adapting-and-preserving-social-science-research/.

Comp, G., Dyer, S. & Gottlieb, M. (2020). Is TikTok the Next Social Media Frontier for Medicine? *AEM Education and Training 5*(3). https://doi.org/10.1002/aet2.10532.

Eghtesadi, M. & Florea, A. (2020). Facebook, Instagram, Reddit and TikTok: A Proposal for Health Authorities to Integrate Popular Social Media Platforms in Contingency Planning Amid a Global Pandemic Outbreak. *Canadian Journal of Public Health = Revue Canadienne de Santé Publique 111* (3), 389–91.

Fullagar, S. & Pavlidis, A. (2021). Thinking Through the Disruptive Effects and Affects of the Coronavirus with Feminist New Materialism. *Leisure Sciences 43* (1–2), 152–9.

Glaw, X., Inder, K., Kable, A. & Hazelton, M. (2017). Visual Methodologies in Qualitative Research: Autophotography and Photo Elicitation Applied to Mental Health Research. *International Journal of Qualitative Methods 16* (1), 1–8.

Haraway, D. (2016). *Staying with the Trouble: Making Kin in the Chthulucene*. Duke University Press.

Harper, D. (2002). Talking About Pictures: A Case for Photo Clicitation. *Visual Studies 17* (1), 13–26.

Hernández, K. J., Rubis, J. M., Theriault, N., Todd, Z., Mitchell, A., Country, B., Burarrwanga, L., Ganambarr, R., Ganambarr-Stubbs, M. & Ganambarr, B. (2020). The Creatures Collective: Manifestings. *Environment and Planning E: Nature and Space 4*(3), 838–63.

Highfield, T. & Leaver, T. (2016). Instagrammatics and Digital Methods: Studying Visual Social Media, from Selfies and GIFs to Memes and Emoji. *Communication Research and Practice 2* (1), 47–62.

Hine, C. (2015). *Ethnography for the Internet: Embedded, Embodied and Everyday*. Bloomsbury Publishing.

Jackson, A. Y. & Mazzei, L. A. (2012). *Thinking with Theory in Qualitative Research*. Taylor & Francis.

Lupton, D. (2019). *Data Selves: More-Than-Human Perspectives*. Polity Press.

Lupton, D., Southerton, C., Clark, M. & Watson, A. (2021). *The Face Mask in COVID Times: A Sociomaterial Analysis*. de Gruyter.

Lupton, D. & Watson, A. (2020). Towards More-Than-Human Digital Data Studies: Developing Research-Creation Methods. *Qualitative Research 21* (4), 463–80.

Mosteanu, O. (2021). City Flows During Pandemics: Zooming in on Windows. In D. Lupton & K. Willis (Eds.) *The COVID-19 Crisis: Social Perspectives* (pp. 53–66). Routledge.

Patterson, A. (2018). YouTube Generated Video Clips as Qualitative Research Data: One Researcher's Reflections on the Process. *Qualitative Inquiry 24* (10), 759–67.

Pink, S., Horst, H., Postill, J., Hjorth, L., Lewis, T. & Tacchi, J. (2015). *Digital Ethnography: Principles and Practice*. SAGE.

Pollitt, J., Grey, E. & Blaise, M. (forthcoming). Enacting a Feminist Pause: Interrupting Patriarchal Productivity in Higher Education. In D. Lupton & Deana Leahy (Eds) *Creative Approaches to Health Education: New Ways of Thinking, Making, Doing, Teaching and Learning*. Routledge.

Priego, E. & Wilkins, P. (2020). Comics as COVID-19 Response: Visualizing the Experience of Videoconferencing with Aging Relatives. *Interactions 27* (4), 60–61.

Rots, A. P. (2017). *Shinto, Nature and Ideology in Contemporary Japan: Making Sacred Forests*. Bloomsbury Publishing.

Silk, M. L. & Andrews, D. L. (2011). Toward a Physical Cultural Studies. *Sociology of Sport Journal 28* (1), 4.

Smith, Aunty S., Smith, N., Daley, L., Wright, S. & Hodge, P. (2020). Creation, Destruction, and COVID-19: Heeding the Call of Country, Bringing Things into Balance. *Geographical Research 59* (2), 160–8.

St. Pierre, E. A., Jackson, A. Y. & Mazzei, L. A. (2016). New Empiricisms and New Materialisms: Conditions for New Inquiry. *Cultural Studies ←→ Critical Methodologies 16* (2), 99–110.

Thomas, J., Barraket, J., Wilson, C. K., Holcombe-James, I., Kennedy, J., Rennie, E., Ewing, S. & MacDonald, T. (2020). *Measuring Australia's Digital Divide: The Australian Digital Inclusion Index 2020*. RMIT and Swinburne University of Technology, Melbourne.

Thorpe, H., Brice, J. & Clark, M. (2020). *Feminist New Materialisms, Sport and Fitness: A Lively Entanglement*. Palgrave Macmillan.

Thorpe, H., Brice, J. & Clark, M. (2021). Physical Activity and Bodily Boundaries in Times of Pandemic. In D. Lupton & K. Willis (Eds.) *The COVID-19 Crisis: Social Perspectives* (pp. 39–52). Routledge.

TikTok. (2020). Privacy Policy. https://www.tiktok.com/legal/privacy-policy?lang=en.

Wang, C. & Burris, M. A. (1997). Photovoice: Concept, Methodology, and Use for Participatory Needs Assessment. *Health Education & Behavior 24* (3), 369–87.

Watson, A., Lupton, D. & Michael, M. (2021). Enacting Intimacy and Sociality at a Distance in the COVID-19 Crisis: The Sociomaterialities of Home-Based Communication Technologies. *Media International Australia 178* (1), 136–50.

World Health Organization. (2020a). #HealthyAtHome. https://www.who.int/campaigns/connecting-the-world-to-combat-coronavirus/healthyathome.

World Health Organization. (2020b). *Novel Coronavirus (2019-nCoV) Situation Report – 13*. World Health Organization, 2 February. https://www.who.int/emergencies/diseases/novel-coronavirus-2019/situation-reports.

11 'Being there' during lockdown: a phenomenological perspective on ethnography of the pandemic present and research methods for the future

L.L. Wynn and Susanna Trnka

Introduction

The COVID-19 pandemic has prompted anthropologists to revisit the discipline's core methodological framework: the assumption that ethnographic research requires us to 'be there' in the field, doing participant observation usually in physical proximity to our research participants and collaborators (and see Southerton, Clark, Watson & Lupton in this collection). During lockdowns and under conditions of public health emergencies around the world, it may not be possible or ethical for us to physically 'be there' in close proximity. Instead, what we are seeing during the pandemic is a complex interdigitation of digital and offline worlds, as people use the Internet to connect with far-flung friends and relatives and incorporate media coverage of global phenomena into their own embodied experiences of COVID-19. In this chapter, we use our own experiences during lockdown in Australia and Aotearoa New Zealand to explore what 'being there' might mean, ranging from digital connections to the use of 'walking ethnography' during lockdown to investigate how people expressed connection, isolation and citizenship while confined to their homes and neighbourhoods. Drawing on phenomenological perspectives, we explore how researchers' own horizons of experience can offer insights into the kinds of research questions and methods that are well suited for exploring research participants' experiences and perceptions while in lockdown. Beyond the pandemic, these methods are important tools for ethnographers to investigate contemporary experiences of isolation, connection and curatorship of online identities in a profoundly digital world.

Lockdown diaries: Sydney, Australia

On Thursday 5 March 2020, Lisa Wynn e-mailed her parents and siblings in the United States and Canada, describing all 22 of the known COVID-19 cases in New South Wales, Australia, which included a staff member at her university, a worker in an aged care facility adjacent to campus and a doctor at the local hospital. She mapped out her house in relation to all the known cases in her state, concluding that she was, literally, located at the epicentre of the pandemic. Her family's biggest concern, she recounted, was the lack of toilet paper in grocery stores.

> Someone posted a news story a week or so ago saying that Australians should stock up on bottled water, TP [toilet paper], long-life milk, and pasta, and that seems to have triggered panic-stockpiling. When I went grocery shopping 2 nights ago, there was literally no long-life milk, no pasta, and not a single roll of toilet paper on the shelves! (Figure 11.1)

She attached to her e-mail the best social media memes about Australia's nationwide toilet paper shortages: pictures of a branch of gum (eucalyptus) leaves hanging from an empty toilet paper dispenser (Instagram, @urntablism-junkies); a toilet paper dispenser loaded with a scarf branded with Aussie Rules football team the Magpies (Instagram, @philpeers); and a tree covered with toilet paper streamers captioned 'Australian government coronavirus response revealed' (Twitter, @obeewhen).

Her brother replied from Las Vegas, where he worked for an amusement park owned by an Australian company, that they had unearthed a box of dust masks in their supply closet, which his colleagues decided were 'like gold.' All the supply companies they usually bought from were completely out of face masks. But, so far, toilet paper was still on shelves in stores. Confidentially, he shared that he was worried about losing his job – and, if he lost his job, he would lose his health-care insurance, a frightening prospect during a pandemic. He would not only be unable to pay his rent but also unable to afford a doctor visit or hospital stay.

Another brother, this one located in Los Angeles, replied saying,

> The local news here in LA is in orange alert/on the brink of panic mode. A health screener at LAX, one of the people whose job it was to identify incoming travellers with symptoms and quarantine them, has tested positive. Then suddenly we started

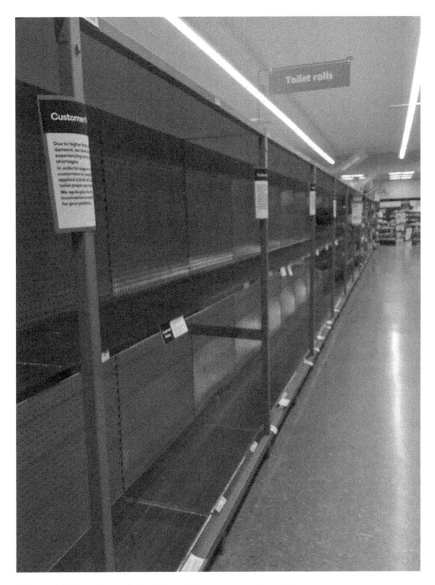

Figure 11.1   No toilet rolls on the supermarket shelves

getting new cases, the mayor declared a state of emergency, and then lo and behold, morons started buying up all the toilet paper. . . . even on Amazon, the freaking toilet paper was on back order. . . . Anyway, that's my report from Los Angeles, the front lines of Armageddon or whatever. Hopefully this apocalypse will pass sooner rather than later so I can wipe my freaking ass.

The next morning, Wynn's sister wrote from Quebec, Canada:

> We've had two cases in Montreal now, so maybe my classes really will be cancelled in a week or two. At this point, we're treating it like snow days.

That night, Wynn got a message from the principal of her children's high school informing parents that there had been a diagnosed COVID-19 case and the school was closing for contact tracing and cleaning. It was the first case of coronavirus in an Australian school. Wynn e-mailed her siblings, informing them that even as her children were ordered to self-isolate her university managers were insisting that she needed to teach her classes in person.

Two hours later, the brother from Las Vegas replied that they currently had eight Aussie executives from the parent company visiting the Las Vegas facility. He had relayed Wynn's report on the Epping Boys High School case and one of the executives immediately excused herself to call her family back in Sydney, some of whom had children at that school. In her COVID-19 diary, Wynn wrote,

> I feel absurdly pleased to have communicated the news to [brother] faster than his Aussie colleagues heard about it. Thus begins the competition amongst all friends and family to share the juiciest tidbits of news before anyone else has heard them.

Correspondence back and forth continued, and on 12 March 2020, Wynn sent her family a link to a blog post by Tomas Pueyo (2020) entitled, 'Coronavirus: Why You Must Act Now' with the comment, 'lots of interesting charts and graphs and info and predictions about coronavirus.' The next day, her father, a geophysicist, replied:

> Lisa, this is the most eye-opening, science-driven analysis I've seen so far. I can actually calculate that 25% of the people in [my workplace] are infected whether they know it or not. I won't be going in anytime soon. THANK YOU. Potentially having up to 480,000 deaths in the USA is absolutely shocking. The 'kill rate' hovering around 40x that of flu is absolutely shocking.

By the end of March, much of Australia was in 'lockdown.' In New South Wales, residents were only allowed to leave their homes for a handful of reasons including to go shopping or to get exercise. Playgrounds were closed (Figure 11.2); shops were plastered with advice about distancing (Figure 11.3). Wynn e-mailed her siblings to tell them that she still had not been able to buy toilet paper.

In her COVID-19 diary entry of 5 April 2020, Wynn wrote,

> [Husband] and I are walking in the evening for exercise and we both simultaneously start to make the same comment: that something has changed in the way we're responding to the pandemic. In the early weeks, we used to wake up every morning

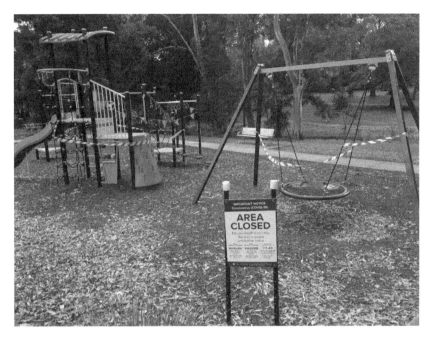

Figure 11.2   Playgrounds closed because of the pandemic

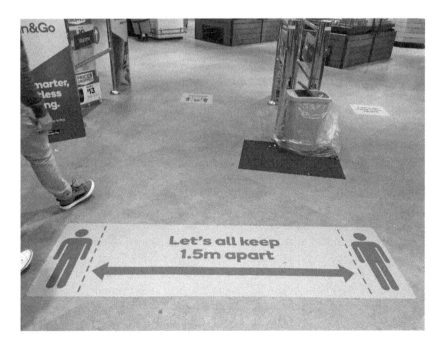

Figure 11.3   Shops instruct on social distancing

and the first thing we'd do before getting out of bed was grab our phones and check the news for new developments: number of reported infections, number of deaths, and for any news about closures (schools, stores and so on) or other laws restricting movement. But our obsessive fixation on the news is easing up.

Reflecting on what had changed, she mused:

> In the beginning, it was both entertainment and felt necessary to find out how much our lives were changing day by day. . . . Why aren't we as obsessively fixated on the news as we used to be? Partly it's that the big changes (school closures, social distancing laws) seem to be fixed in place and haven't changed significantly for a week or two. Partly it might just be news fatigue. But then [husband] commented, 'There's something about exponential growth. It's very exciting. And it's not exponential anymore.'

Two months later, Australia experienced its second, deadliest 'wave' of COVID-19 infections. Infections and deaths were an order of magnitude beyond what they had been before. Exponential growth fixed their attention on the news again. Every morning began with rolling over in bed, grabbing the phone from its charger, and opening a local news website to find out what the new death toll was.

* * *

This brief glimpse into how one Australian academic experienced the first few months of the COVID-19 pandemic tells us a lot about how the pandemic played out in Sydney (with glimpses of Los Angeles, Las Vegas, and Montreal) and the pressing concerns of people as they were living through it: a relentless scanning of headlines; a fixation on case numbers and locations; e-mails to check in on faraway family and friends; relating novel states of emergency with familiar ones (snow days); using humour to make sense of social responses to the pandemic; sharing memes on social media (particularly memes with local takes on the global pandemic); armchair epidemiology, as people sought knowledge about a mysteriously novel pathogen and its implications; walking the neighbourhood in the evenings for exercise and to escape the confines of home during lockdown; counting deaths. Minor inconveniences (toilet paper shortages) juxtaposed with the fear of major life changes (job loss and the precarity of access to healthcare) shape a sense of an unprecedented historical moment mediated by humour ('the front lines of Armageddon or whatever') and digital connection. It tells a story about how knowledge is gained and circulated, and about the horizons of knowledge (Merleau-Ponty, 2010; Ram & Houston, 2015). Public health information was filtered through online newspapers and television broadcasts, social media, family and friends.

These selections from a pandemic diary also offer us a challenge and an opportunity to think about the present and future of ethnographic research, not just in times of a pandemic. For anthropologists, sociologists, geographers and other social scientists who use ethnographic methods to understand the world, participant observation is the sine qua non of qualitative methods. Being with people allows us to understand how they move through the world, share knowledge and reproduce and challenge cultural norms, generating insight that clinical experiments never can; participant observation shows us the differences between what people *say* they do (in interviews, for example) and what they *actually* do; ethnography contextualises statistical and survey data to show what population-level trends mean at the level of individual lived experience.

But how do we do ethnographic research during a pandemic? When the government has mandated that we all stay home, or only socialise within our own 'bubble,' how can we *be there* with those outside of our bubble? How do we grasp the day-to-day lives of others, much less begin to understand their responses to previously unheard of government directives?

Qualitative research in the midst of social and political instability has the potential to reveal social, political and ethical fault lines that might in other circumstances be more easily obscured (Greenhouse, 2002). That said, research conducted in the midst of a pandemic must be attuned to local circumstances – the ethical implications of asking interlocutors to reflect on their experiences by filling in a survey or partaking in Zoom interviews during lockdown in Aotearoa New Zealand (where actual levels of COVID-19 infections have remained comparatively extremely low), are, for example, quite different than doing so in India, Brazil, or the United States, but nonetheless require careful reflection (Rogers, 2021).

The horizons of our own pandemic experiences show our limitations as researchers, but they also suggest important questions to ask about our research participants' experiences and understandings of the pandemic. In this chapter, we draw on the insights of phenomenology to map out the possibilities and limitations of ethnographic research during the COVID-19 pandemic. In the process, we sketch the parameters of contemporary ethnographic research methods, not only during the pandemic but beyond.

'Being there': an imaginary baseline

From the earliest years of the discipline, anthropologists have prioritised 'being there' with our research participants in order to understand their lives on their own terms. The British-trained Polish anthropologist Bronislaw Malinowski is often credited with being the father of the ethnographic research method, after spending two years in the Trobriand Islands, an archipelago off the east coast of what is now Papua New Guinea, living with the natives. He described that experience in several books, including his most famous, *Argonauts of the Western Pacific* (1922), and his most infamous (until the posthumous publication of his diaries): *The Sexual Life of Savages* (1929), which described the erotic lives of the Trobrianders. It was in *Argonauts* that Malinowski laid out his argument for an ethnographic research method. To adequately understand and describe another culture, the anthropologist must 'grasp the native's point of view, his [sic] relation to life, to realize his vision of his world' (Malinowski, 1922, p. 25). At nearly the same intellectual moment of the early twentieth century, Franz Boas was leading the development of American anthropology with a similar philosophy of field research, centring around his concept of 'cultural relativism': the idea that people's actions, beliefs, and moral codes made sense only within the context of their own cultural norms and belief systems. It was thus the job of the anthropologist to spend extended periods of time in that culture, learn its language, participate in everyday life and collaborate with local informants (who were at once research participants, native researchers, and guides) in order to grasp others' actions and moral worlds. Boas's most famous student, Margaret Mead, implemented this method in her influential *Coming of Age in Samoa* (1928).

The principles of participant observation, extended residence and learning the local language advanced by Malinowski, Boas, Mead and others soon became the hallmarks of the ethnographic research method, combined with other qualitative methods including interviewing, charting kinship relations and mapping village life and resource extraction. Ethnography became, in short, a matter of 'being there' – a phrase so core to the method that it that has been the title of more anthropological elaborations of research methodology than we can possibly list, from books like Bradburd's (1998) *Being There: The Necessity of Fieldwork* to Watson's (1999) *Being There: Fieldwork in Anthropology* to Borneman and Hammoudi's (2009) *Being There: The Fieldwork Encounter and the Making of Truth* to Davis and Konner's (2011) *Being There: Learning to Live Cross-Culturally*, not to mention countless journal articles and book chapters. For a century, *being there* has been 'the central ritual of the [anthropological] tribe' with its accompanying mythology (Stocking, 1983, p. 70).

Even when the phrase has been used to subvert traditional formulations of ethnographic field methods (for example, in Hannerz's [2003] reflection on multi-sited anthropology, 'Being there . . . and there . . . and there!'; in Lennartsson's [2011] formulation of a historical ethnographic agenda, 'Notes on 'not being there''; or in Angelone's [2019] 'Virtual ethnography: The post possibilities of not being there'), the phrase works to establish co-presence as the default against which all other methodological approaches must define and justify themselves. And even as ethnography has become the province of multiple disciplines and anthropology has moved away from its tradition of single-sited village ethnographies to write about transnational scientists and online worlds, the ideal of co-presence continues to inform methodological approaches, from Traweek's ethnography of high-energy particle physicists eating in the cafeteria together (1988) to Rabinow's hanging out in a genetics lab to study the scientists of polymerase chain reactions (1996) to Boellstorff's ethnography of a virtual world (2008) in which he argued that anthropologists of online spaces could still *be there* with their research participants.

How can we 'be there' with our research participants during quarantine and lockdown? What are the implications of conducting fieldwork 'at a distance' (Käihkö, 2020)? While the pandemic has undoubtedly been a rupture unlike anything that has come before it, with cities around the world confining citizens in strict lockdowns, it has nevertheless highlighted the changing nature of ethnography in a digital era, regardless of pandemic status. Even while trapped in our own homes and neighbourhoods, most of us remained radically globally connected via technology to friends, family, colleagues and research participants – connections that long predated pandemic physical distancing. COVID-19 lockdowns thus offer us a lens for thinking about how to understand contemporary forms of connection and dislocation, rupture and continuity, that have characterised pandemic experiences and beyond.

In this chapter, we use accounts of our fieldwork during COVID-19 lockdowns in Sydney and Auckland, Aotearoa New Zealand to explore the reach and the limits of ethnography in times of pandemic. We approach this from the perspective of phenomenology and the idea that the task of ethnographers is to document our research participants' horizons of perception, within the limitations of the researchers' own horizons. We explore how the concept of horizons can encompass the ways that people interact on- and offline to shape temporalities and hybridities, focusing on the ways that people's consumption of media, government messaging and stories of others' experiences moulds, and is moulded by, their own lived realities to create a complex interdigitation of online spaces and embodied offline experiences.

Lockdown diaries: Auckland

The day Aotearoa New Zealand entered into nationwide lockdown, anthropologist Susanna Trnka stood in her bedroom in West Auckland feeling a rising sense of panic. Whilst cognisant that she was extremely privileged to have a house that feels safe and comfortable, and to be part of a family she was happy to lockdown with, she could not bear the thought that for at least the next 28 days, her world would be encompassed by the same four walls. She grabbed her walking shoes and decided to take up the Prime Minister's invitation to leave home for the purposes of exercising in one's neighbourhood. How far, she wondered, does one's neighbourhood extend? Could it perhaps be as far as they can comfortably walk? And how far is that? She walked about 2.3 kilometres until she could glimpse the sea, repeating it the next day, and the next, until it became a daily ritual.

On her walks, she not only ruminated over her own embodied experience of lockdown, considering carefully the sensation of walking and how simply moving through space gave her a sense of connection to others (past, present and future), but also took note of what those she encountered during her daily journeys were doing. Some scenes were hard to forget: a man in a garden chair strategically placed outside of his home was listening to an old-fashioned transistor radio belting out Hindi devotional songs, as if to build a sonic wall that separated him not only from passers-by, but the other members of his residence. Although closed, the local golf course seemed to have attracted locals desperate for a secluded space for quiet reflection. Others were less unusual – people walking on the street instead of on the sidewalk to ensure physical distancing; children playing on playgrounds despite closure signs – but nonetheless had much to say about people's reactions to the pandemic and to lockdown.

Much like an ethnographer who has just entered a new field site and has not perhaps completely mastered the local language, she found herself scanning people's movements, comportment, gait and even eye contact in public places, as clues for interpreting sociality. Ethnographers have long noted that how we occupy public space is shaped by gender, class, age and ethnicity (for example Newcomb, 2009). Now we can add fears of contagion and attitudes towards lockdown regulations to the list, watching whether passers-by decide to impose a much greater distance than two metres between themselves and anyone else on the sidewalk or who decides to sit on park benches in contravention of level 4 lockdown rules.

People's bodies emit signs available for interpretation (Foucault, 1991), as do material objects. Houses, for example, speak of their owner's or occupiers' lives. We can read their outsides (as well as insides), learning about their occupants from such characteristics as modes of adornment, arrangement of objects and attentiveness (or not) to contemporary fashions (Miller, 2008). At the start of lockdown, Aotearoa New Zealand's Prime Minister publicly endorsed the Teddy Bears in Windows movement which aimed to communicate 'hope' and

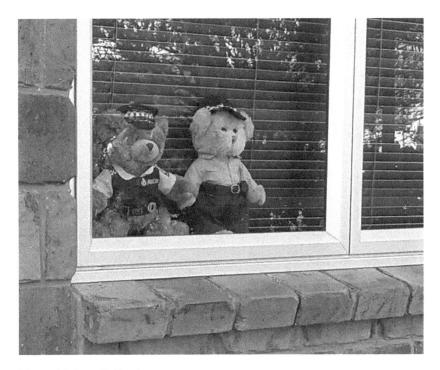

Figure 11.4   Police bears

'care' to others by means of the display of children's teddy bears in residential windows. Within the first week of her walking ethnography, Trnka noticed house after house in her predominantly working class, West Auckland neighbourhood had put together, often elaborate, formations of bears and other stuffed animals or figurines in their front windows, on porches or in some cases, tied onto lampposts outside their homes (Figure 11.4, see also Trnka, 2020a). Some were explicitly marked to align with government messaging, such as stuffed animals in plastic bags bearing the words 'be kind,' or 'be safe & look after your friends.' A few were seemingly subversive in intent, such as sunbathing bear, stretched out on a beach towel, wearing a bikini beside a cold drink and sunblock (at a time when anyone actually doing so on the beach would've been contravening level 4 restrictions), and two bears dressed up in police uniforms, appearing to surveil, as much as reassure, the passing public (Figure 11.5).

Desperate to know what was going on outside of her neighbourhood, Trnka asked her adult child who lives in another major urban area to send photos of house fronts so she could determine if the Teddy Bear displays there looked substantially

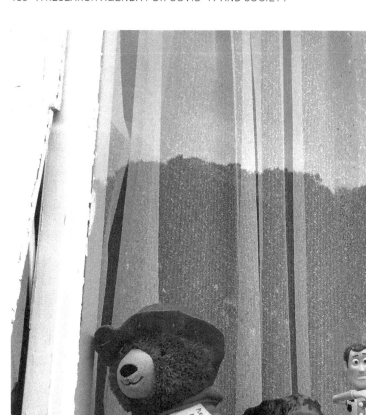

Figure 11.5   Bear in window

different (Figure 11.4) (they didn't). At level 3 when regulations enabled 'staying regional' (rather than just local), she undertook 'drive-by ethnography' (Levine & Manderson, 2021) of other areas in the city, and when lockdown levels eased even further, she ventured further afield, photographing leftover signs and stuffed animals as evidence of community responses during previous alert levels.

Documenting the Teddy Bears in Windows phenomenon as well as the other ways that public space was both symbolically recast and physically inhabited demonstrates how ethnography can continue to take place even when mobility is limited. Obviously watching people move through public space or taking photographs of their homes can only tell us so much; but when coupled with physically distanced methods of participant observation of social media or response to mainstream reporting (that is, reading online comments boxes or Reddit discussion groups), or direct questioning about other people's experiences and perspectives through online surveys, phone interviews or Zoom discussions, it can be a vital facet in, for example, developing an understanding of New Zealander's affective and embodied responses to government directives.

Methodological extensions and limitations

In the midst of various kinds of lockdowns, ethnographers around the world have drawn from a range of resources to continue practicing their craft. These include auto-ethnography in the form of personal, daily reflections on their experiences in a COVID-19 diary (as Wynn undertook), or daily postings on social media intended to prompt dialogue and discussion with other researchers (as Trnka did). Visual diaries – whether one's own or those of participants – can take many forms, including photography, video, drawings or citizen science initiatives which enable participants to upload images or use maps to reflect on their lockdown experiences. In a similar vein, ethnographers can prompt first person accounts by encouraging our interlocutors to make digital diaries or reflective recordings (Clark, 2020). More 'traditional' methods of engaging with participants can also be conducted online, such as Zoom or WhatsApp interviews, online surveys or participant observation in online forums, be they academic conferences, 'zui' (hui taking place over Zoom) or talanoa around virtual kava bowls (Fehoko et al., 2021).[1]

Obviously, however, such engagements do not allow for spending a full day, or days on end, following around one's interlocutors – a hallmark of classic, ethnographic research. And there are other limitations. Research drawing from social media must account for how algorithms structure not only our own feeds but those of our interlocutors (cf. Cheney-Lippold, 2011), making it even more imperative to carefully document people's sources of news and information, the social media platforms they use, how and when they use them as well as the friends and family they are in contact with.

Living through lockdown, perhaps more than ever, we are limited in our ability to access the lives of those whose experiences are radically different to ours. Wynn's experiences of walking around her middle-class suburban Sydney neighbourhood told her little about what it's like to be unemployed and living in inner city Redfern, or an elderly person living in an aged care facility and barred from physical contact with the outside world, or a farmer in the Outback simultaneously experiencing COVID-19 lockdown while recovering from the 2019–20 bushfires. Trnka found that her students who lived in the next neighbourhood recounted feeling higher levels of discomfort when moving through public spaces as they were concerned over potentially drawing the attention of the police due to previous experiences of racism, gender violence, and class prejudice (see also Aikman, 2020). Without pre-existing relationships of trust with people, it may become even harder to connect outside our own 'bubbles' as we become physically confined in our own neighbourhoods and homes. One of the key tenets of 'being there,' that is, standing alongside our interlocutors to better ascertain their positionality, has become even more of a struggle.

Just as with interviews, we are, moreover, limited by what information people choose to share with us. How do we measure what people say against what people do if we are not there to witness the doing? Will the pictures and stories that people share of life under lockdown be as carefully curated as their social media profiles? And, of course, we can have little insight into the lives of those who are less digitally connected, either due to lack of access or very limited access because of financial barriers, or those who find themselves in situations, such as domestic violence, or the breakdown of romantic or kin relationships, that they do not wish to speak about with others. All of these are aspects of crisis ethnography that should not stop our research endeavours, but rather, must be accounted for in the findings and interpretations we present.

A phenomenology of lockdown: our horizons of perception

A phenomenological approach to the ethnographic method seeks to document the horizons of people's experience, knowledge and belief. Ram and Houston (2015, p. 1) define phenomenology as 'an investigation of how humans perceive, experience, and comprehend the sociable, materially assembled world that they inherit at infancy and in which they dwell . . . phenomenology . . . sets out to show how experience and perception are constituted through social and practical engagements.' Phenomenology has often been applied to studies of illness and healing, embodiment, sociality and senses of place (Desjarlais & Throop, 2011), all of which are of particular relevance to understanding pandemic experiences. Indeed, the body is at the core of philosopher Maurice Merleau-Ponty's framing of perception in terms of horizons: that which determines all that we experience and understand of the world, including the not just the scope of our perceptions and experience but also the limitations of what we perceive, know and experience (Merleau-Ponty, 2010).

In the context of COVID-19, this phenomenological approach might in part attend to temporalities of the pandemic. We might ask questions about futurity: how are people imagining the horizons of our future in the wake of a global crisis? How do imaginations of future horizons (lockdowns, releases from lockdowns, a future availability of toilet paper, the development of a vaccine, the future opening of borders and resumption of travel, etc) inform how we live in the present (and see Goode's chapter)?

We might also examine horizons of the past: how do we come to experience an epidemic as a rupture with the past (cf. Briggs & Mantini-Briggs, 2004)? Looking back on the past year of pandemic and lockdown, what do people remember most vividly about pandemic experiences? How might their initial experiences of the crisis manifest today, as embodied traces, sensory memories and/or discursive accounts? These are questions we have been asking in our own research on pandemic experiences. In both responses to online surveys and in qualitative interviews, what is striking is how people's responses meld media coverage, government messaging and personal experiences: something they read in the newspaper leads them to formulate an understanding of the state's role in our private lives; the social media posts they read inform their understandings of what constitutes acceptable and unacceptable protocols for social interactions during the pandemic; an epidemiological forecast shared by e-mail between family members shapes their thinking about government policy responses. We also find how the re-shaping of the mundane quotidian experiences of daily life – waking up, going through the day, passing evening after evening during lockdown – can recast their understandings of what a satisfactory or meaning-filled life can look like. Several New Zealand respondents remarking that the lockdown granted them, in one woman's words, a greater sense of 'perspective on what's most important in life' (Trnka et al., 2021). Others have felt burdened by the strain of intensified inter-connectivity, inciting desires for greater separation from those with whom they've been forced to share lockdown (cf. Strong et al., 2021).

Our analyses of these responses lead us to the question of hybridities of experience and perception. During lockdowns, many of us have turned to the various mediations of the Internet to understand what was happening outside of our own homes and neighbourhoods. How are people incorporating media coverage, social media memes and humour, government policies, epidemiological forecasting and biologists' pronouncements about invisible forces into their individual and social experiences? How do media and government catch phrases become part of their own distinct stories? Phenomenology examines the mediation of experience and perception to describe 'phenomena as they appear to the consciousness of certain people' (Ram & Houston, 2015, p. 4). We propose that in a pandemic era, this 'mediation' might particularly attend to how *media* (including social media, news broadcasts, epidemiological charts, government press conferences and so on) act as interface between our immediate embodied experiences and our perceptions of a pandemic as an abstract concept about a local, regional, national or global phenomenon.

There are always limits to ethnographers' ability to phenomenologically grasp other people's experiences, knowledge and beliefs. Despite traversing through the same spaces and embodying similar lifeworlds, we may not be able to experience grief, loss, rage and other emotions in the same way as our research participants (Das, 2006; Rosaldo, 1980; Trnka, 2020b). Cultural taboos may prevent us from being able to document the sensual and affective dimensions of other people's erotic, sexual experiences (Wynn, 2018) and other intimate forms of life that cultural norms dictate are shameful or private or for other reasons not to be shared widely. People's experience may include that which is unconscious, unspeakable or beyond the grasp of language (Das, 2006; Ram & Houston, 2015; Trnka, 2008). Yet a phenomenological approach to ethnography fully accounts for these limitations, because it recognises that even as we (researchers) seek to understand and describe other people's horizons, we are limited by our own horizons of perception. We are not only documenting lockdown experiences, we are living them, too – living through the very phenomena we are documenting and having our own affective responses to them. We experience the fear, or thrill, of lockdown, the panicked recognition of having been in the same shop or bus as the latest 'case' whose 'locations of interest' are being broadcast on the radio, or the concern over how and when to have a COVID-19 test, or access a vaccine. Similar to ethnographers who work in situations of disaster, national revolution or political violence (Greenhouse, 2002; Trnka, 2008), the 'field' is not a space from which we can easily extract ourselves; we are both researcher and participant in this pandemic in ways we cannot escape.

This phenomenological perspective on the limitations of research is consonant with the insights of feminist and 'halfie' (Abu-Lughod, 1991) anthropology and the literature on embodiment: whatever we know, we know through our own bodies, including our physical appearance, dis/ability, gender, age, ethnicity, socioeconomic background, education, accent and dialect and language spoken and so on. All of these shape not only our understanding of the world but also the way our research participants interact with us, what they perceive our research agendas to be and what kinds of information they share or exclude from conversations. Knowledge is always partial. Perception, as Edmund Husserl (2012) showed us, is always dependent on our positioning in the world. By moving through time and space, towards objects and towards one another, we can attempt to gain a different vantage point (Patočka 1998). Ethnography is one way of conceptualising and enacting such movement (Trnka, 2020b). It is not fool proof, nor is it meant to be. What is vital is that we recognise that and seek to sketch out not only the ways that our own knowledge remains partial but also why we and others find ourselves located as we do.

Conclusions: mapping out an agenda for future ethnographic research post-pandemic

Malinowski made necessity a virtue when he was interned in the Trobriand Islands during WWI for two years; forced by the war and his Polish citizenship to spend an extended period of time with the Trobrianders (which was at the time colonised by the British), he recognised the methodological value of long-term engagement and participant observation of the lives of his research participants. We can make necessity a virtue, too: experiences of simultaneous isolation and connectedness during the pandemic take to an extreme what anthropologists have been observing for years about how our worlds are changing and its implications for ethnographic research methods.

The pandemic itself is a global phenomenon as are our attempts to mitigate and end it whilst also sustaining social life in its midst. Ethnographic research is in many ways a quotidian practice, based on the depths of understanding gained through hour after hour of engagement, whose aim is to interpret the mundane as well as the sensational in the unfolding lives of our interlocutors. Thrust by global crises into similar conditions as those whose 'everyday' experiences (of life in the midst of a pandemic) we aim to interpret, we must tread a careful line between extrapolating from our own experiences and perceptions, documenting those of others and remaining acutely cognisant of the limits of this enterprise. Not to do so would be disingenuous. Not to do so would be to lose a historic opportunity to understand how the COVID-19 crises that unfold around us are likely to dramatically re-shape lifeworlds for generations to come. A phenomenological approach to pandemic and post-pandemic social worlds seeks to document the horizons of people's perceptions and experience in a globally interconnected world, while at the same time recognising the methodological limits of our own horizons as researchers.

Note

1   Hui is a Māori term for a gathering, meeting or assembly. Talanoa is a Pacific term denoting inclusive, participatory dialogue, and can refer to anything from a formal discussion to an informal chat. Both terms are commonly used in Aotearoa New Zealand.

References

Abu-Lughod, L. (1991). 'Writing Against Culture.' In Richard Fox (Ed.), *Recapturing Anthropology: Working in the Present* (pp. 137–62). Santa Fe, NM: School of American Research Press.

Aikman, P. J. (2020). 'Partnership is Crucial during a Crisis.' *E-Tangata*. May 24. https://e-tangata.co.nz/comment-and-analysis/partnership-is-critical-during-a-crisis/

Angelone, L. (2019). 'Virtual Ethnography: The Post Possibilities of Not Being There.' *Mid-Western Educational Researcher 31*(3), 275–95.

Boellstorff, T. (2008). *Coming of Age in Second Life: An Anthropologist Explores the Virtually Human.* Princeton University Press.

Borneman, J. & Hammoudi, A. (Eds.) (2009). *Being There: The Fieldwork Encounter and the Making of Truth.* Berkeley, Los Angeles: University of California Press.

Bradburd, D. (1998). *Being There: The Necessity of Fieldwork.* Smithsonian Institute.

Briggs, C. L. & Mantini-Briggs, C. (2004). *Stories in the Time of Cholera: Racial Profiling During a Medical Nightmare.* University of California Press.

Cheney-Lippold, J. (2011). 'A New Algorithmic Identity: Soft Biopolitics and the Modulation of Control.' *Theory, Culture & Society 28*(6), 161–81.

Clark, M., (2020). 'Digital Diaries as Social Research Method.' https://www.youtube.com/watch?v=xRuxXp-ud54&t=114s

Das, V. (2006). *Life and Words: Violence and the Descent into the Ordinary.* University of California Press.

Davis, S. H. & Konner, M. (2011). *Being There: Learning to Live Cross-Culturally.* Cambridge: Harvard University Press.

Desjarlais, R. & Throop, J. (2011). 'Phenomenological Approaches in Anthropology.' *Annual Review of Anthropology 40*, 87–102.

Fehoko, E., Hafoka, 'I. & Tecun, A. (2021). 'Holding Tightly onto Land and People During a Pandemic: Kava Pedagogies and Tertiary Learning Relationships in Vahaope.' *Journal of Global Indigeneity 5*(1): 1–15. https://www.journalofglobalindigeneity

.com/article/19432-holding-tightly-onto-land-and-people-during-a-pandemic-kava
-pedagogies-and-tertiary-learning-relationships-in-vahaope

Foucault, M. (1991). *Discipline & Punish: The Birth of the Prison*. Translated by Alan Sheridan. Vintage.

Greenhouse, C. J. (Ed.) (2002). *Ethnography in Unstable Places: Everyday Lives in Contexts of Dramatic Political Change*. Duke University Press.

Hannerz, U. (2003). 'Being There . . . and There . . . and There!: Reflections on Multi-Site Ethnography.' *Ethnography* 4(2), 201–16.

Husserl, E. (2012). *Ideas: General Introduction to Pure Phenomenology*. Translated by W. R. Boyce Gibson. Routledge.

Käihkö, I. (2020). 'COVID-19, Ebola, and the Ethnographic Distance.' *Items: Insights from the Social Sciences*. 6 August. https://items.ssrc.org/covid-19-and-the-social-sciences /social-research-and-insecurity/covid-19-ebola-and-the-ethnographic-distance/

Lennartsson, R. (2011). 'Notes on 'Not Being There': Ethnographic Excursions in Eighteenth-Century Stockholm.' *Ethnologia Europaea* 41(1), 105–13.

Levine, S. & Manderson, L. (2021). 'Proxemics, COVID-19 and the Ethics of Care in South Africa.' In *'L'enfer, c'est les autres': Proximity as an Ethical Problem During COVID-19*, T. Strong, S. Trnka & L. L. Wynn (Eds.), *Cultural Anthropology* 36(3):391–9.

Malinowski, B. (1922). *Argonauts of the Western Pacific*. Dutton.

Malinowski, B. (1929). *The Sexual Life of Savages in North-Western Melanesia*. Routledge & Kegan Paul, Ltd.

Mead, M. (1928). *Coming of Age in Samoa*. William Morrow and Co.

Merleau-Ponty, M. (2010). *Phenomenology of Perception*. Translated by D. A. Landes. Routledge Classics.

Miller, D. (2008). *The Comfort of Things*. Polity.

Newcomb, R. (2009). *Women of Fes: Ambiguities of Urban Life in Morocco*. University of Pennsylvania Press.

Patočka, J. (1998). *Body, Community, Language, World*. Translated by E. Kohák & J. Dodd (Ed.). Open Court.

Pueyo, T. (2020). 'Coronavirus: Why You Must Act Now.' *Medium*, 10 March. https://medium.com/@tomaspueyo/coronavirus-act-today-or-people-will-die -f4d3d9cd99ca

Rabinow, P. (1996). *Making PCR: A Story of Biotechnology*. Chicago University Press.

Ram, K. & Houston, C. (2015). 'Introduction: Phenomenology's Methodological Invitation.' In K. Ram & C. Houston (Eds.), *Phenomenology in Anthropology: A Sense of Perspective* (pp. 1–28). Indiana University Press.

Rogers, D. (2021). 'Resuming Field Research in Pandemic Times, Redux: A View from Inside a "Research Reactivation" Committee.' *Items: Insights from the Social Sciences*, 6 May. https://items.ssrc.org/covid-19-and-the-social-sciences/social -research-and-insecurity/resuming-field-research-in-pandemic-times-redux-a-view -from-inside-a-research-reactivation-committee/

Rosaldo, M. (1980). *Knowledge and Passion: Ilongot Notions of Self and Social Life*. Cambridge University Press.

Stocking, G. W. Jr. (1983). 'The Ethnographer's Magic: Fieldwork in British Anthropology from Tylor to Malinowski.' In G. Stocking (Ed.) *Observers Observed: Essays on Ethnographic Fieldwork* (pp. 70–120). University of Wisconsin Press.

Strong, T., Trnka, S. & Wynn, L. L. (Eds.). (2021). ''L'enfer, c'est les autres': Proximity as an Ethical Problem During COVID-19.' *Cultural Anthropology* 36(3), 341–9.

Traweek, S. (1988). *Beamtimes and Lifetimes: The world of High Energy Physicists.* Harvard University Press.

Trnka, S. (2008). *State of Suffering: Political Violence and Community Survival in Fiji.* Cornell University Press.

Trnka, S. (2020a). 'From Lockdown to *Rāhui* and Teddy Bears in Windows – Initial Responses to COVID-19 in Aotearoa/New Zealand.' *Anthropology Today 36*(5), 11–13.

Trnka, S. (2020b). *Traversing: Embodied Lifeworlds in the Czech Republic.* Cornell University Press.

Trnka, S. et al. (2021). 'Negotiating Risk and Responsibility: Affect and Ethical Reasoning in New Zealanders' Lived Experiences of Lockdown.' *Journal of the Royal Society of New Zealand 51*(Issue sup. 1): S55–S7. http://dx.doi.org/10.1080/03036758.2020.1865417

Watson, C. W., (Ed). (1999). *Being There: Fieldwork in Anthropology.* Pluto Press.

Wynn, L. L. (2018). *Love, Sex, and Desire in Modern Egypt: Navigating the Margins of Respectability.* University of Texas Press.

12 'Normal was a problem' – post-pandemic futures

Luke Goode

Introduction

Will historians look back on this pandemic as a catalyst that shifted the world onto a new track? Will it appear retrospectively as a pivotal crisis that spurred governments to make good on their promises to 'build back better,' one that energised communities and social movements to organise for the common good on an unprecedented scale? Or will it read as yet another miserable chapter in the history of disaster capitalism: corporate profiteering; deepening divisions and inequalities; and global leaders furnished with new alibis for their chronic failure to respond adequately to the climate catastrophe unfolding before their eyes?

The answer will surely be more complex than the question implies: like prior pandemics (Hays, 2005; McNeill, 1998), this one will shape history in ways we cannot foresee. But as far as our naïve question is meaningful, the answer future historians will give depends substantially on the ways in which governments, parties, activist movements, corporations, citizens and communities act (or choose not to act) in this moment of amplified risk and opportunity.

The crisis is still unfolding. The sands have been shifting from the start and, even once it is declared 'over,' its impacts will reverberate in complex ways for a long time to come.[1] As Matthewman's chapter in this volume makes clear, it is neither wise nor particularly useful to try and predict how COVID-19 will shape the future while we are still in its midst (and for further meditations on futurity see Trnka and Wynn's chapter). In this chapter, however, I am less concerned with the pitfalls of making specific and concrete *predictions*. Instead, I'm interested in a more general phenomenon, namely, the very terrain on which 'the future' is envisioned and contested. From the early days of this pandemic—even as the world was scrambling to understand and respond to the nature and scale of this new threat—the terms on which a world *after* COVID-19 could be envisioned were already being contested. Did the arrival of this new crisis open up new vistas of social possibility? Could it be an unprecedented opportunity to remake the world? Or was the challenge instead to find the best pathway back to pre-COVID-19 normality?

The future is not simply a site for idle speculation but an imaginative and discursive terrain upon which political projects, policies and corporate strategies are built, as well as the aspirations and expectations of everyday citizens. The capacity to shape public expectations about the future is a form of political power. That power lies not simply in persuading people this or that prediction is likely to 'come true' but in defining the future as a horizon of possibilities: what types of future are desirable and, even more fundamentally, what types of future are actually thinkable to begin with.

Crisis and discursive contestation

On the one hand, then, the pandemic has been framed as a rupture, exposing new possibilities (Milne et al., 2020); an event that has made it easier to imagine different and better ways of being. It has allowed some critical distance from ingrained social, cultural and economic habits, encouraging reflection on deficiencies of the preceding 'situation normal.' This has manifested at micro-levels of everyday life. We have glimpsed what cities can look like when the traffic and smog clear (Young et al., 2021). Workers who have been furloughed or able to work remotely have tasted different rhythms of everyday life. For many workers, of course, it has been a time of heightened pressure rather than enhanced autonomy and wellbeing that has provoked reflection on the meanings and experiences of work—the 2021 'great resignation' wave in the United States (Kamal, 2021) reflects changes in the labour market but perhaps also signals a broader cultural shift in attitudes towards work (Parker et al., 2020; Richardson & Klein, 2021). This notion that the pandemic has created valuable distance from and encouraged critical reflection on prior normalities also registers at other scales: we have seen community initiatives flourishing—some aimed at feeding the hungry, others simply at keeping spirits up. And we've seen international leaders (Joe Biden, Boris Johnson and Jacinda Ardern among them) adopting 'Build Back Better' rhetoric, sensing public preferences for change over a speedy return to business as usual.

Such shifting sentiments are reflected in various in opinion surveys. In 2020, for example, an IPSOS survey of 21 000 adults across twenty-seven countries found 86 per cent 'want the world to change significantly and become more sustainable and equitable rather than returning to how it was before COVID-19' (Boyon, 2020). But we should be careful what we wish for: public appetites for change represent an opportunity for powerful elites, as much as for progressive forces. As it happens, that survey was commissioned by the World Economic Forum (WEF), the collective mouthpiece of the Davos global elite. WEF openly describes the pandemic as a 'rare but narrow window of opportunity to reflect, reimagine, and reset our world' (WEF, 2020) in its own undemocratic, although increasingly green-washed, image (Wecke, 2021).

On the other hand, rather than a catalyst for transformation, the pandemic has been framed with equal if not greater fervour as a deeply inconvenient interruption to business as usual. In this frame, concerns are voiced about the mental health harms of protracted lockdowns and restrictions as well as the moral legitimacy of limiting individual freedoms. Loudest of all, however, are concerns about economic damage and calls for these to be properly weighed against public health risks. Business lobbies, political leaders and media outlets—although less so, ordinary citizens (Lazer et al., 2020, p. 6)—invoke the economic damage argument as if it were an obvious common sense imperative to return to 'normality,' that is, to fully re-open markets, international borders, shops, workplaces and ancillary service industries as soon and fully as possible. The qualifier 'as possible' raises many troubling questions. What rates of death, severe illness and health system strain are acceptable? What value should we place on the lives of those who are most at risk from relaxing public safety measures? Is this a matter of moral reasoning or a simple cost–benefit calculus (Spinney, 2021; The Economist, 2021a)? These are questions that cheerleaders for a speedy return to 'normality' prefer not to have to confront (Devlin, 2021).

The Economist has established a pandemic 'normalcy index,' ranking countries by how closely life there has returned to a 'baseline of what global normality looks like' (2021b), using indicators like traffic volumes and retail footfall. They acknowledge some things will never be the same again. However, the normativity is clear: restoring pre-pandemic levels of monetary and human mobility is to return to a desirable normality, a natural state of affairs. While *The Economist* has never hidden its ideological commitment to globalised market capitalism,[2] normality discourse also enjoys a more pervasive reach, manifesting in less overt ways. Pew Research, for example, conducted a survey in March 2021 asking Americans how long they believe it will be before 'businesses, schools, places of worship operate about as they did before the COVID-19 outbreak,' with a majority of respondents saying they expected it would be at least one to two years or longer (Dunn, 2021). In Pew's survey report, this is interpreted as low public 'optimism.' Linguistic slippage rather than evidence of an ideological agenda, perhaps, it nonetheless illustrates how the desirability of returning to pre-COVID-19 normality becomes a default assumption wherever it is not explicitly questioned. The onus is on those who would question its desirability; on those who would remind us that 'normality' was already a privileged rather than universal condition prior to the pandemic (see Lambert's chapter in this volume); and on those who would argue that the pre-COVID-19 world was already 'post-normal' (Sardar, 2010).

Stated briefly, then, my interest lies in this tension: the pandemic as a time of potentially enhanced media and public receptivity towards re-imagining the future, towards reassessing what is taken to be 'normal' or 'inevitable,' and potentially even towards genuinely transformative politics; offset against a powerful drive to return to a pre-pandemic 'normality,' however phantasmic that may be. The latter is propelled by powerful vested interests but, as the pandemic rolls on, it can increasingly capitalise on the anxiety and fatigue of citizens enduring a prolonged period of uncertainty. How, then, should we understand this apparent tension and what might it tell us about the prospects for social and political transformation?

I want to suggest some basic contours of a research agenda framed around this question. But some qualifiers are necessary beforehand. First, I do not claim this tension is unique to this particular moment. Disasters and crises are commonly sites for competing frames emphasising new possibilities opened up in their wake, on the one hand, and prioritising recovery of what has been lost on the other (Guggenheim, 2014). Secondly, in no sense is the coexistence of two rhetorically opposed frames (roughly 'build back better' versus 'back to normal') in itself reflective, let alone constitutive, of a social contradiction. We should even be cautious about characterising these as being in tension without first digging below surface-level rhetoric.

'Build back better' has a particular contextual and institutional (although not uncontentious) history in the development of key principles for inter-national disaster recovery programmes, including an emphasis on empow-ering local communities to be active authors of their own future (UNDRR, 2015). But this has not prevented 'build back better' from becoming an expedient floating signifier in the context of domestic politics, embraced by political leaders who can be described as moderate technocratic reformers at best and are largely committed to defending the status quo. Depending on context, speaker and intended audience, 'build back better' can mean piecemeal increases in public health funding and more public–private partnerships with pharmaceutical companies to bolster preparedness for future pandemics. But it can also signal something more transformative:

policies to address the structural inequalities that ensured already vulnerable and disenfranchised communities have suffered the impacts of COVID-19 most severely (Godfery, 2021; Martin, 2021). In the United States, Biden has tabled legislation dubbed the 'Build Back Better' bill[3] comprising policies such as modest increases in child tax credits, some improvements in health insurance affordability, promises to 'strengthen the middle class' through more affordable housing and education, and 'better preparing the nation for future pandemics and supply chain disruptions' (The White House, 2021). Is it transformative? Define 'transformative.'

In 2020, with the pandemic in full swing around the world, New Zealand's Labour Party, led by Jacinda Ardern, secured a record election victory. 'Build back better' was a campaign slogan. Putting an economic regeneration spin on the concept, the campaign publicity highlighted job creation and apprenticeship programmes, infrastructure spending and regional investment (NZ Labour, 2021). In a speech to chief executive officers at the 2020 Asia-Pacific Economic Cooperation summit (a major annual meeting of government and business leaders in the Asia-Pacific region), Ardern gave the phrase 'build back better' an altogether less Keynsian gloss, emphasising instead economic growth through global trade as the key to a brighter future: 'As we confront this generation's biggest economic challenge, we must not repeat the mistakes of history by retreating into protectionism. APEC must continue to commit to keeping markets open and trade flowing.' Ardern highlighted Digital Economy Partnerships with Chile and Singapore as evidence of New Zealand's commitment to 'build back better' (APEC, 2021). Define 'transformative.'

The competing 'back to normal' frame is also subject to substantial slippage. Invoking the need for a return to 'normality' can equally play to corporate interests desperate to see consumers fully back in shopping malls or workers back in office blocks, *and* to fundamental human needs and desires for more social interaction and engagement with the outside world. So while the drive for normalcy may unreflectively evoke a return to prior routines of work and consumption, it may also provoke reflection on the very meaning of 'normal,' that is, on which aspects of life before COVID-19 have been most sorely missed and are therefore most highly valued.

As a communication researcher, I focus heavily on discourse, language and rhetoric, but not because these are proxies for material and structural realities. Communication research typically explores how language conceals and obfuscates as much as it reveals. But while it may be depressing to witness these slippery frames exploited for political expediency, this semiotic indeterminacy may also signal a space of possibility, a discursive terrain amenable to contestation. Greenpeace New Zealand, for example, has taken up Ardern's embrace of the 'build back better' slogan as its own critical yardstick, articulating its criticisms of the government in terms of the latter's failure to meet the standards it has rhetorically committed itself to (Larsson, 2020). This one localised example is not presented as evidence for any generalisable trend but simply to illustrate that those with the greatest power to shape the narrative are never guaranteed to fully control where their rhetoric leads; and nor, by extension, the terms under which publics perceive the boundaries of what is (im)possible or (un)realistic.

Identifying 'build back better' and 'back to normal' as two master frames speaks to my particular interest in *futures* discourse. Both are explicitly temporal frames, figuring respectively an orientation towards social change and an orientation towards restoration of a prior state. I will have more to say about the intersection between communication and futures research in the following section. But one further qualifier is required before proceeding. I am not suggesting that these master frames should be exclusive points of focus. There are other significant frames that, while not explicitly temporal in nature, shape the discursive constitution and contestation of possible futures and which are significant in the pandemic context. Two aspects in particular are especially pertinent: discursive framings of 'society' and 'value.'

The discursive constitution of society manifests most obviously in popular discourse through the invocation of a collective 'we.' Often media and political discourses appeal to shared interests and circumstances, addressing themselves to or purporting to speak on behalf of an imagined community. Who comprises that imagined community is routinely assumed rather than stated or questioned. Drawing on another example from my home country, PM Ardern received widespread positive coverage in international media during earlier phases of the pandemic for her communicative skill in evoking a sense of common national purpose. In particular, her repeated references to the 'team of 5 million' in her appeals for lockdown compliance (and later, vaccination uptake) was a key weapon in her rhetorical arsenal (Beattie & Priestley, 2021). As the pandemic has developed, especially with uneven vaccination rates leaving already disenfranchised communities at greatest risk, there has been growing criticism of the gap between the universal rhetoric and the highly unequal reality (Daalder, 2021). The government's own strategy has also shifted, recognising that messages shaped by and for specific communities and demographics are critical, and that it is untenable to assume a diverse and highly unequal population will cohere around national figureheads just because they adopt an inclusive and empathetic style of communication (Ioane et al., 2021; Thaker, 2021).

In New Zealand, COVID-19 has also prompted debate and reflection around social cohesion. One line of analysis emphasises how important high levels of social cohesion are to the management of the crisis (Spoonley et al., 2020). Another sees the fact that divisions and inequalities have become more visible as the crisis progresses as an illustration of the urgent need to reassess what 'social cohesion' actually means (Lewis & Morgan, 2021). In this view, dominant conceptions focus heavily on public sentiment and government rhetoric (emphasising tropes of togetherness, inclusion and kindness). This serves an ideological role in papering over entrenched structural and material inequities and 'feeds into an unhelpful (and unhealthy) "COVID nationalism"' (p. 4). Stated briefly, both perceptions and realities of social cohesion, and the way these have been impacted by the pandemic, have profound implications for the range of possible futures that could be built in the wake of COVID-19.

The way social value is framed in popular discourse is also important. Put simply, we need to ask whether the pandemic has disrupted dominant perceptions of what value *is* and which social actors are its key creators. The dominant neoliberal ideology of Anglo-American democracies views economic value created through profit-seeking (mythically fuelled by competition, innovation and entrepreneurial spirit) as the root of all social value. The pandemic, however, has led governments around the world to act in ways that very visibly contravene neoliberal common sense, including major stimulus spending and re-socialising parts of the economy. It remains to be seen whether this will mark a sustained shift toward 'strategic state-building' in Anglo-American democracies (Mishra, 2020) and expanded social license for 'Big Government' initiatives beyond the immediate crisis, a prospect that is clearly alarming the economic Right (Bourne, 2021). But the crisis clearly represents a moment of expanded possibility: an environment in which citizens and enterprises most visibly depend upon the state to keep them safe is one in which demands for truly transformative policies that would significantly (re)socialise the economy can, in principle, appear less 'radical,' less 'dangerous,' more 'realistic.' Besides state agency, media discourses during the pandemic have also amplified the value created by other non-corporate actors including community organisations and previously undervalued workers in health and other frontline occupations. Will this pandemic mark a period of intensified and sustained societal reflection on the meaning of social value, on what constitutes socially valuable work, and on toxic notions of productivity? Or will the drive to restore normalcy ensure there is no lasting damage to neoliberal common sense? The answer will shape the horizon of possible futures that can be imagined, demanded and created in the wake of the pandemic.

Communicating futures

My current research focus straddles two inter-disciplinary fields: Communication and Futures Studies. Communication programmes and departments are commonplace across universities internationally and the field has become established over many decades. Futures Studies is less widely known, however. And while I have studied Communication over the course of three decades, I have only engaged with the Futures field during the past few years, having been only dimly aware of its existence prior to that. It exists as a named field in relatively few academic institutions and is often misunderstood as being wholly pre-occupied with prediction and forecasting, as a field closely aligned to strategic planning in military and/or corporate spheres, or as dubious pop futurology dressed up as if it were serious social science.

Recounting the lengthy and complex history of the Futures field is beyond the scope of this chapter (see Bell, 2003; Gidley, 2017; Sardar, 2013), but a very brief sketch is useful before going further. Futures Studies focuses on the ways in which social actors (including individuals, communities, organisations and institutions) envision, articulate, contest and shape the future. The use of 'futures' in the plural underscores that the point is not to correctly forecast *the* future—to bet on the right horse, as it were—but to study, using various methodologies and conceptual frameworks, the ways in which potential futures are continually subjected to social shaping and contestation. This is not to fall into the idealist trap of thinking the future is somehow infinitely open—indeed, the Futures field also explores processes through which societies, communities and organisations become locked into particular pathways, and by which alternative possible futures become closed off (Adam & Groves, 2007). That future generations are already locked into dangerous levels of climate change is the starkest of examples. Nonetheless, the notion that the future is neither fully knowable nor pre-determined is a central axiom of, rather than an inconvenient obstacle to, research in the Futures field.

The plural form of 'futures' is significant for other reasons too. Futures researchers study how people, groups and institutions think and act with reference to various timescales, from decades to centuries to epochs. They also engage with and highlight diverse (though inter-related) social scales that frame our engagements with the future: at the micro-level of individual life plans; at the scale of communities and organisations planning for the future; through to beliefs about the future of the human species and the planet. Importantly, the cultural and historical shaping of temporalities, that is, different ways of thinking about time and about the relationships between past, present and future, also comes into play. Although some strains of Futures research have been guilty of unreflexively reproducing Eurocentric assumptions, critical work in the field problematises and decentres linear views of time and 'progress' associated with Western colonial modernity, bringing in diverse cultural perspectives (Gidley, 2017, pp. 56–9).

In the remainder of this chapter, I will highlight two primary dimensions of research located at the intersection between Communication and (critical) Futures Studies. Specifically, I aim to do so in a way that speaks to some of the key issues raised by the COVID-19 pandemic. In short, the first dimension (Hegemonic Futurism) engages with debates, ideas and beliefs that explicitly address 'the future,' that is, it interrogates the ways in which the future is *articulated*. By contrast, the second (Discounted Futures) interrogates ways in which the future is *silenced*. While both dimensions have a critical and diagnostic orientation, each also brings a reconstructive dimension into play (Goode & Godhe, 2017), inviting researchers to explore how the problems identified might be addressed in practice. The brief sketch below is necessarily incomplete, and the examples I give are highly selective, intended only to indicate an emergent research agenda rather than provide a definitive map.

Hegemonic futurism

This dimension is about confronting dominant narratives of the future. It questions who enjoys the greatest power, legitimacy and influence in articulating visions of the future. In short, self-styled 'futurists' and corporate 'thought leaders' are vastly over-represented in this space as go-to sources for popular media seeking expert insights into what the future may hold (Goode, 2020). Corporate leaders, especially from the digital technology sector, not only wield some of the most powerful voices articulating visions of the future, but also have enormous material resources and power at their disposal to shape the future in alignment with their visions and their interests. This dimension of analysis also interrogates the substance of hegemonic narratives. What are these 'futurists' actually saying about the future when we dig beneath the surface? What are they *not* saying—for example, about the huge carbon footprint, extractive economies and labour exploitation underpinning their high-tech visions? While hegemonic futurism routinely narrates its techno-centric visions in terms of the future of 'humanity,' this dimension of analysis requires us to deconstruct this presumed 'we' and question who would actually thrive and who would suffer in the kind of future being projected by corporate leaders like Jeff Bezos and Elon Musk (Murtola, 2018) or by popular pundits of the future like Yuval Noah Harari (2016) who reinforce these techno-centric narratives, even as they avoid explicitly advocating for them.

Silicon Valley futurism has become such a dominant perspective over recent decades in part because of the vast resources at its disposal: it is a well-funded arm of the tech sector's public relations strategy, designed to persuade policy makers and the wider public that the industry is uniquely placed to furnish the world with solutions to humanity's grand challenges (Morozov, 2013). But Silicon Valley futurism has also been able to flourish because, under neoliberalism, institutional politics has largely abandoned the project of long-term imagination in favour of economic managerialism (Fisher, 2009; Mulgan, 2020). Ambitious, transformative political programmes founded on positive visions of the future have been successfully villainised as impractical and dangerous utopianism, while corporate and techno-centric visions have enjoyed unrivalled power to shape popular future imaginaries (Jasanoff & Kim, 2015).

In the coming few years it will be interesting to observe whether the Silicon Valley worldview continues to exert the same influence over popular imaginings of the future. In the years leading up to the pandemic, disquiet about the concentrated power and corporate ethics of large technology behemoths including Facebook, Alphabet (Google) and Amazon was already growing in volume, becoming increasingly prominent in mainstream media and political discourse. During the pandemic itself, we had the grotesque spectacle of Bezos, Musk and Richard Branson ramping up their pitiful competition to lead a new corporate space race. The UN Secretary General was provoked to condemn these 'billionaires joyriding in space while millions go hungry on Earth' (Guterres, 2021), and no less an establishment figure than the heir to the British throne was also moved to get in on the act, condemning them for throwing their money at the space race in the midst of a climate emergency (Bowden, 2021). None of this should lead us to presume the pandemic will mark a tipping point from which the cultural power of tech billionaires starts waning: they continue to enthuse and inspire substantial armies of wide-eyed followers. But when ardent scepticism takes root in the mainstream and even among elite powers, their continued status as premier definers of the future is not guaranteed.

The mere possibility of chinks in the armour starting to appear would also raise the possibility of increased opportunities for alternative, more equitable, sustainable and human rather than techno-centric visions for the future (Gidley, 2017, pp. 100–15) to gain a stronger foothold in the public sphere. But the issue is not simply whether hegemonic futurism per se may be waning in influence, but also whether we may see it mutating over coming years. One plausible scenario is that the brand of tech futurism promoted by the likes of Musk and Bezos will at some point 'read the room' and try to re-brand itself with a greener gloss. And we've already noted the example of the Davos elite using this pandemic to promote their own grand vision for the future: a 'Great Reset' which will supposedly create 'a healthier, more equitable, and more prosperous future' (WEF, 2020).[4] So the forms and loci of hegemonic futurism may shift and critical researchers will need to be watching this space.

The privileged status of techno-centric worldviews in shaping popular imagination about the future over recent decades is not simply an isolated function of the rising power of the tech industry, nor does it simply reflect trends in futures forecasting. It also has to be understood in the wider context of a neoliberal project which has, particularly in Anglophone societies, conferred on capitalist interests a powerful aura of legitimacy in defining the needs, priorities and values of society more generally. It is possible, although by no means certain, that corporate leaders will have to negotiate a more crowded field of authoritative voices and perspectives in the wake of the pandemic. Preceding the pandemic, declining trust in professional expertise was an increasingly prominent concern (Nichols, 2017). Indeed, COVID-19 has created new vectors for mistrust, from vaccine scepticism to outright conspiracy theories of a manufactured crisis. Yet it has also amplified the public visibility of experts including epidemiologists, data modellers and professional science communicators, with surveys indicating heightened levels of trust in scientists (Spoelstra, 2020; see also Sibley et al., 2020). Professional scientists, in contrast to corporate thought leaders, less readily trade in grandiose prognostications. But any sustained elevation of trust and popular interest in public (that is, not corporate-aligned) science raises at least the possibility of a shift in mainstream media habits towards consulting a broader range of expert voices to inform debates about the long-term direction of society. Unfortunately, such an outcome is not only far from certain; we should also be realistic about how transformative it could be. Elevated public trust in scientific expertise does not necessarily rub off on *social* scientists (Boswell, 2021), less still *critical* social scientists, even though socially grounded perspectives on the future are vital. Importantly, too, there are significant issues around representation and diversity in the range of scientific expert voices centred by mainstream media during the pandemic (Greaves, 2021).

As previously indicated, the challenge for researchers in this space is not simply to diagnose the symptoms and causes of the narrow range of voices dominating public discourse about the future. The challenge is also to explore avenues for redress. In the wake of the pandemic, the challenge is to understand the current moment as a space of change and uncertainty, and therefore as a space of possibility—although one at risk of rapidly dissipating in the push to resuscitate 'normality.' A research agenda for post-pandemic futures must urgently address how to diversify the range of ideas and perspectives on the future in ways that will have popular reach. Part of this entails mainstreaming and popularising ideas that are already out there but are currently invisible to or not considered serious or 'realistic' by a majority of lay citizens: for example, proposals relating to universal welfare, workplace democracy, public or community ownership of infrastructure, the digital commons or reimagining democracy to give voice to future generations (Krznaric, 2020, pp. 163–93). And it means exploring and developing concrete proposals for ways of diversifying the voices informing public debates about the future—not only widening the range of *expert* insights but also proposals to amplify lay voices from diverse backgrounds in order to treat citizens as 'experts in their own tomorrows' (Raven, 2020).

Discounted futures

My discussion of hegemonic futurism might prompt the following question: does the way Jeff Bezos (or any other billionaire) thinks and speaks about the future matter nearly so much as his immense financial power? (Conversely, does giving 'voice' to marginalised perspectives on the future matter nearly so much as the access to the material resources citizens require to be active agents in shaping their own futures?) I'd argue both matter, but it is true that the degree of control that powerful interests exert over the future rests on accumulations of power that may have little or nothing to do with explicitly articulated visions of the future designed to captivate popular imagination. So is that a distracting side-show? Mainstream media have covered the issue of pandemic profiteering, whereby corporations like Amazon have exploited the crisis to cement their market dominance, while US billionaires, including Bezos, collectively increased their personal fortunes by 70 per cent in just 19 months (Collins, 2021). But news of this sort does not rival the attention-grabbing power of a spectacle like Bezos, dressed as a space cowboy, launching a nonagenarian Captain Kirk into low orbit (Koren, 2021), even though its implications for the future may be more profound. Nor does it lend itself as readily to debates about the long-term implications (besides rather superficial speculation about whether Bezos will become the world's first trillionaire) compared to a publicity spectacle explicitly framed in terms of what it augurs for 'the future.'

From a communication perspective, this is not simply an exercise in throat clearing designed to ward off materialist objections. Rather, it highlights a communicative deficit that needs to be properly diagnosed and urgently confronted. Public debates about the future tend to be triggered by narratives explicitly announcing themselves as views on the future, especially those produced by self-styled futurologists and corporate thought-leaders. Popular media are awash with content labelled 'The Future of X' (for example work, energy, artificial intelligence, space exploration, education, medicine and so on) framed by expert insights and futuristic visions of the powerful. Exceptional occurrences—financial crashes, pandemics, extreme weather events, global summits on climate change or tech billionaire publicity stunts—can also trigger moments of reflection and debate about the future. But the public sphere is extremely ill-equipped to foster democratic debate and reflection on the structural, institutional and everyday processes already embedded in the present that are quietly yet profoundly shaping the future possibilities that lie ahead.

The political economy of today's mediascape, combined with ingrained cultural assumptions about what constitutes 'newsworthy' content, ensures our public sphere is event-driven and obsessed by the exceptional and spectacular. Yet any hopes of limiting the power of elites to determine the future behind our backs rest in no small part on building a public sphere that critically interrogates not only explicit hegemonic *visions* of the future, but also the ways in which our 'normal' ways of doing things have created such vast disparities of power and put the future of the entire planet in the hands of so few. Even when billionaires cash in so handsomely on the exceptional circumstances created by the pandemic, including the suffering and deaths of millions, the news is liable to stir only temporary anger and disgust, rather than burning itself into our eyeballs as it probably should. Perhaps future historians will look back and wonder why that story was not sufficient to incite a popular movement for public reappropriation of billionaire wealth. But from the vantage point of today, while there is something excessive and distasteful about the story, there is nothing exceptional in elites exploiting exceptional circumstances. It is ostensibly 'normality' on speed. So while democratic deliberation about the future requires critical engagement with ideas *about* the future, it also depends on our capacity to de-normalise the normal. Currently, however, most of our media and political institutions are at best ill-equipped for this and, at worst, actively work against it.

Debates about 'the future' are marked out as a special category of public discourse, a momentary zooming out from our presentist default. For the most part, however, the production, consumption and discussion of news and current affairs proceeds as if there is no future beyond the next electoral or economic cycle, or beyond the current crisis; and it proceeds largely as if there are no future generations. 'Discounting the future' is a financial and moral sleight of hand used in mainstream economics to treat the harms caused by today's (in)actions as being less 'costly' the further into the future those harms will be suffered (Weisbach & Sunstein, 2009). But it is also an apposite term for a more general condition of the contemporary public sphere, one that has severe consequences for society's capacity to address the challenges before us in anything like a democratic, deliberative fashion.

Besides pandemic profiteering, COVID-19 has given rise to a range of issues with potentially significant long-term implications, ones that are liable to be discounted unless they are subject to sustained critical attention. One example is the risk of surveillance creep, were digital tools designed to manage a major public health emergency to become quietly normalised and find applications beyond the exceptional remit for which they were designed and originally implemented. The risk is heightened by the role that governments have given to profit-driven tech corporations in the development and deployment of these tools (Roberts, 2020). The potential long-term consequences for mental health of the COVID-19 crisis is another issue of global relevance (WHO, 2021). Another key area of concern is the prospect of structural inequalities becoming more firmly entrenched in the wake of the pandemic, condemning already disadvantaged groups to an even tougher future than the one they already faced. In New Zealand, for example, some immediate impacts of the pandemic on Māori are clear enough: Māori are substantially over-represented in case numbers, hospitalisations and deaths (Jacobs, 2021), and most at risk from the relaxation of public health restrictions (McLure, 2021a; Steyn et al., 2021) (for an expanded discussion of COVID-19's impact on Indigenous populations see Lambert in this collection). But there are also serious concerns about long-term impacts, from shifts in the labour market caused by the pandemic that threaten to disrupt an entire generation of young Māori (BERL, 2020), to evidence that the New Zealand government's housing policy during the pandemic has 'baked in Māori inequality for generations' (White, 2021). One final but stark example: delays to action on climate change attributed to the pandemic (Tollefson, 2021). The crisis has of course presented some real challenges—according to New Zealand's Climate Minister, for example, progress on a critical emissions reduction policy stalled because it was impossible during lockdown to conduct meaningful consultation with communities most likely to be affected by the transition (RNZ, 2021). The long-term risk, of course, is that a precedent has been set and each new major emergency (be it subsequent pandemics or even emergencies generated by climate change itself) provides another reason to kick the can further down the road.

The problem is not that the long-term implications of these issues have not received any attention whatsoever in mainstream public discourse during the pandemic. Rather, it is the prospect that what limited debate they have generated will rapidly dissipate as attention shifts elsewhere. The challenge is to consider how these issues and their long-term implications might be kept in the spotlight and how we avoid them receding into the background to become part of a 'new normal' that is even more toxic than the one that prevailed before this crisis.

The communication deficit as I've framed it here—failure in our public sphere to properly debate the potential long-term consequences of things that have occurred in the midst of crisis—not only threatens to obscure the true scale of risks and harms. It also risks missing the opportunity to debate and build on some potentially *positive* developments when these are framed only as an ephemeral artefact of exceptional times. Could proposed changes to intellectual property arrangements around pharmaceuticals not only assist in the fight against COVID-19 but also potentially lay the groundwork for longer-term reforms that would shift the global public health landscape in a more equitable direction (Gurgula & Lee, 2021)? In New Zealand, there have been unprecedented levels of partnership between police and Indigenous communities (Stanley & Bradley, 2020) and even between local 'gangs' (largely demonised in the past in mainstream media and political discourse) and public health officials (McLure, 2021b). Could this become a springboard for sustained and positive social change? Will the fact that the NZ government was suddenly in a position to provide shelter for every homeless person during the first wave of the virus (Donavan, 2020) shift societal perceptions of what is possible and realistic when there is sufficient political will? Or are these examples destined to pass into the history books as exceptional occurrences dictated by exceptional circumstances? With these positive phenomena, the challenge is reversed: to keep them in the communicative spotlight, to avoid discounting their potential to shape the long-term future, to hold open the possibility that they *do* in fact become part of a 'new normal,' one that is *less* toxic than the normality that prevailed before.

Conclusion

What I have attempted to sketch out here, in provisional and incomplete fashion, is a general direction for a research agenda located at the intersection of Communication and Futures Studies, one that can address in a limited but meaningful way the urgent imperative to minimise the long-term harms and injustices wrought in the wake of this pandemic. Framed in more constructive and ambitious terms, it might even contribute towards reframing the pandemic as a 'rare and unique opportunity' – for motives resolutely different from those of the World Economic Forum, of course. In case this seems glib, there is no claim being made here that COVID-19 has suddenly gifted us the opportunity of a bright new future. As I write this conclusion, it is hard enough to imagine the end of COVID-19, let alone the end of capitalism. But the pandemic has stirred things up, and our capacity as a society to explore new possibilities depends significantly on the conversations and debates we have about them, and whether these conversations and debates can be sustained over time.

During the pandemic, I was struck by an image of a masked Greenpeace protester holding a sign that read: 'Normal was a problem. Future can be better.' It struck me as both absurd and profoundly depressing. The statement seems so blindingly obvious that it should not even need to be said. And yet it needs to be said. One way to think about the challenge ahead might be to ask ourselves what it would take for such a statement to assume its rightful place as basic common sense such that it no longer needs spelling out and the focus of our conversations can shift from *whether* a better future is possible to concentrate instead on the question of *how*.

Notes

1   See Dittmer & Lorenz's discussion of the 'pandemocene' in this volume.
2   It has also sought to reassure its readership that the 'Great Resignation' does not amount to any real shift in cultural attitudes towards work or materialist values (The Economist, 2021c).
3   At the time of writing, this is widely deemed unlikely to pass through Senate.
4   WEF's 'Great Reset' has fuelled right-wing conspiracy theories about a global communist takeover. In case it is not totally clear, this bizarre take is not one I share.

References

Adam, B. & Groves, C. (2007). *Future Matters: Action, Knowledge, Ethics.* Brill.
APEC (2021). 'Prime Minister Jacinda Ardern Talks with Microsoft President Brad Smith.' https://www.apec2021nz.org/apec-nz-2021/apec-news/prime-minister -jacinda-ardern-talks-with-microsoft-president-brad-smith.
Beattie, A. & Priestley, R. (2021). 'Fighting COVID-19 With the Team of 5 Million: Aotearoa New Zealand Government Communication During the 2020 Lockdown.' *Social Sciences and Humanities Open* 4(1), 1–10.
Bell, W. (2003). *Foundations of Futures Studies Volume 1: History, Purposes, and Knowledge.* Routledge.
BERL. (2020). 'Ka Whati te Tai: A Generation Disrupted.' Māori Futures Collective. https://knowledgeauckland.org.nz/media/1954/challenges-opportunities-maori-post -covid-19-ka-whati-te-tai-berl-april-2020.pdf.

Boswell, C. (2021). 'COVID-19 Has Increased Trust in Science: Can It Do the Same for the Social Sciences?' London School of Economics. https://blogs.lse.ac.uk/impactofsocialsciences/2021/08/27/covid-19-has-increased-trust-in-science-can-it-do-the-same-for-the-social-sciences/.

Bourne, R. (2021). 'The COVID-19 Case for Bigger Government Is Weak.' *Pandemics and Policy*. Cato Institute.

Bowden, G. (2021). 'Prince William: Saving Earth Should Come Before Space Tourism.' *BBC News*, 14 October. https://www.bbc.com/news/uk-58903078.

Boyon, N. (2020). 'How Much Is the World Yearning for Change After the COVID-19 Crisis?' IPSOS. https://www.ipsos.com/sites/default/files/ct/news/documents/2020-09/global-yearning-for-change-after-the-covid-19-crisis-2020-09-ipsos.pdf.

Collins, C. (2021). 'U.S. Billionaire Wealth Surged by 70 Percent, or $2.1 Trillion, During Pandemic.' Institute for Policy Studies. https://ips-dc.org/u-s-billionaire-wealth-surged-by-70-percent-or-2-1-trillion-during-pandemic-theyre-now-worth-a-combined-5-trillion/.

Daalder, M. (2021). 'The Stark Inequality of the Vaccine Rollout.' *Newsroom*, 6 September. https://www.newsroom.co.nz/the-stark-inequity-of-the-vaccine-rollout.

Devlin, H. (2021). 'Why Britons Are Tolerating Sky-High COVID Rates – and Why This May Not Last.' *The Guardian*, 15 October. https://www.theguardian.com/world/2021/oct/15/why-britons-are-tolerating-sky-high-covid-rates-and-why-this-may-not-last.

Donavan, E. (2020). 'Clearing the Streets of Rough Sleepers.' *The Detail* (podcast). *Radio New Zealand*, 30 June. https://www.rnz.co.nz/programmes/the-detail/story/2018752191/clearing-the-streets-of-rough-sleepers.

Dunn, A. (2021). 'A Majority of Americans Expect It Will Be At Least a Year Before Life Returns To the Way It Was Before COVID-19.' *Pew Research Center*. https://www.pewresearch.org/fact-tank/2021/03/11/a-majority-of-americans-expect-it-will-be-at-least-a-year-before-life-returns-to-the-way-it-was-before-covid-19/.

The Economist (2021a). 'How to Assess the Costs and Benefits of Lockdowns.' *The Economist*, 3 July. https://www.economist.com/finance-and-economics/2021/07/01/how-to-assess-the-costs-and-benefits-of-lockdowns.

The Economist (2021b). 'COVID-19: When Will Life Return to Normal?' *The Economist*, 8 July. https://www.economist.com/films/2021/07/08/covid-19-when-will-life-return-to-normal.

The Economist (2021c). 'Evidence for the 'Great Resignation' Is Thin On the Ground.' 11 December. https://www.economist.com/finance-and-economics/evidence-for-the-great-resignation-is-thin-on-the-ground/21806659.

Fisher, M. (2009). *Capitalist Realism: Is There No Alternative?* Zero Books.

Gidley, J. (2017). *The Future: A Very Short Introduction*. Oxford University Press.

Godfery, M. (2021). 'By Ending COVID Elimination, Jacinda Ardern Once Again Fails to Turn Compassion into Policy.' *The Guardian*, 5 October. https://www.theguardian.com/world/commentisfree/2021/oct/05/by-ending-covid-elimination-jacinda-ardern-once-again-fails-to-turn-compassion-into-policy.

Goode, L. (2020). 'Hegemonic Futurism and Popular Debate.' In A.M. Murtola & S. Walsh (Eds.) *Whose Futures?* (pp. 35–55). Economic and Social Research Aotearoa.

Goode, L. & Godhe, M. (2017). 'Beyond Capitalist Realism: Why We Need Critical Future Studies.' *Culture Unbound* 9(1), 108–29.

Greaves, L. (2021). 'Māori Experts Have Been All but Invisible in the Government COVID-19 Response. Why?' *The Spinoff*, 7 October. https://thespinoff.co.nz

/politics/07-10-2021/maori-experts-have-been-all-but-invisible-in-the-government
-covid-19-response-why.

Guggenheim, M. (2014). 'Introduction: Disasters as Politics—Politics as Disasters.' *The
Sociological Review 62*(S1), 1–16.

Gurgula, O. & Lee, W.H. (2021). 'COVID-19, IP and Access: Will the Current System
of Medical Innovation and Access to Medicines Meet Global Expectations?' *Journal
of Generic Medicines 17*(2), 61–70.

Guterres, A. (2021). 'Secretary-General's Address to the 76th Session of The UN
General Assembly.' United Nations. https://www.un.org/sg/en/node/259283.

Harari, Y.N. (2016). *Homo Deus: A Brief History of Tomorrow*. Harper.

Hays, J.N. (2005). *Epidemics and Pandemics: Their Impacts on Human History*.
ABC-Clio.

Ioane, J., Percival, T., Laban, W. & Lambie, I. (2021). 'All-of-Community by All-
of-Government: Reaching Pacific People in Aotearoa New Zealand During the
COVID-19 Pandemic.' *The New Zealand Medical Journal 134*(1533), 96–103.

Jacobs, M. (2021). 'One Hundred Days of Harsh Lessons for Māori as Calls for
Help Go Largely Unanswered.' *Stuff*, 25 November. https://www.stuff.co.nz/pou
-tiaki/300460675/one-hundred-days-of-harsh-lessons-for-mori-as-calls-for-help-go
-largely-unanswered.

Jasanoff, S. & Kim, S. (Eds.) (2015). *Dreamscapes of Modernity: Sociotechnical
Imaginaries and The Fabrication of Power*. University of Chicago Press.

Kamal, R. (2021). ''The Great Resignation': June's US Jobs Report Hides Unusual
Trend.' *The Guardian*. https://www.theguardian.com/business/2021/jul/03/us-jobs
-report-june-trend.

Koren, M. (2021). 'Jeff Bezos Is Being Knocked Back Down to Earth.' *The Atlantic*,
2 October. https://www.theatlantic.com/science/archive/2021/10/jeff-bezos-blue
-origin-toxic-workplace-allegations/620279/?utm_source=feed.

Krznaric, R. (2020). *The Good Ancestor: How to Think Long Term In A Short-Term
World*. Penguin.

Larsson, A. (2020). 'Five Ways NZ Will Be Much Better if Jacinda Makes Good on Her
Promise to Build Back Better.' Greenpeace Aotearoa. https://www.greenpeace.org
/aotearoa/story/five-ways-new-zealand-great-jacinda-ardern-promise-build-back
-better/.

Lazer, D., Baum, M.A., Ognyanova, K. & Volpe, J.D. (2020). 'The State of the
Nation: A 50-State COVID-19 Survey.' COVID-19 Consortium. https://osf.io/arwh3
/download.

Lewis, N. & Morgan, J. (2021). 'Trouble with Social Cohesion: The Geographies and
Politics of COVID-19 in Aotearoa New Zealand.' *New Zealand Geographer*, 1–4.
https://doi.org/10.1111/nzg.12314.

Martin, H. (2021). 'Lessons To Be Learnt from COVID-19 Hitting Auckland's Most
Vulnerable.' *Stuff*, 1 October. https://www.stuff.co.nz/national/health/coronavirus
/300419277/lessons-to-be-learnt-from-covid19-hitting-aucklands-most-vulnerable
--experts.

McLure, T. (2021a). 'Māori Party Warns Reopening New Zealand Amid COVID
Outbreak Would Be 'Modern Genocide.'' *The Guardian*, 11 October. https://www
.theguardian.com/world/2021/oct/11/maori-party-warns-reopening-new-zealand
-amid-covid-outbreak-would-be-modern-genocide.

McLure, T. (2021b). 'Unusual Bedfellows: How Gangs Are Pushing New Zealand's
COVID Vaccination Drive.' *The Guardian*, 21 November. https://www.theguardian

.com/world/2021/nov/21/unusual-bedfellows-how-gangs-are-pushing-new-zealands
-covid-vaccination-drive.

McNeill, W.H. (1998). *Plagues and Peoples*. Anchor Press.

Milne, S., Hendricks, C. & Mahanty, S. (2020). 'From Bushfires to Coronavirus, Our Old 'Normal' Is Gone Forever. So What's Next?' *The Conversation*, 9 April. https://theconversation.com/from-the-bushfires-to-coronavirus-our-old-normal-is-gone-forever-so-whats-next-134994.

Mishra, P. (2020). 'Flailing States.' *London Review of Books* 42(14). https://www.lrb.co.uk/the-paper/v42/n14/pankaj-mishra/flailing-states.

Morozov, E. (2013). *To Save Everything, Click Here: The Folly of Technological Solutionism*. Public Affairs.

Mulgan, G. (2020). 'The Imaginary Crisis (and How We Might Quicken Social and Public Imagination).' *Demos*. https://demoshelsinki.fi/julkaisut/the-imaginary-crisis-and-how-we-might-quicken-social-and-public-imagination/.

Murtola, A.M. (2018). 'How The Global Tech Elite Imagine the Future.' *Economic and Social Research Aotearoa*. https://esra.nz/global-tech-elite-imagine-future/.

Nichols, T. (2017). *The Death of Expertise: The Campaign Against Established Knowledge and Why It Matters*. Oxford University Press.

NZ Labour (2021). 'Building Back Better.' 23 July. https://www.labour.org.nz/news-building_back_better_2021.

Parker, K., Horowitz, J. & Minkin, R. (2020). 'How the Coronavirus Outbreak Has—and Hasn't—Changed the Way Americans Work.' *Pew Research Center*. https://www.pewresearch.org/social-trends/wp-content/uploads/sites/3/2020/12/PSDT_12.09.20_covid.work_fullreport.pdf.

Raven, P.G. (2020). 'Experts in Their Own Tomorrows: Placemaking for Participatory Climate Futures.' In C. Courage et al. (Eds.) *The Routledge Handbook of Placemaking* (pp. 148–58). Routledge.

Richardson, N. & Klein, S. (2021). 'People at Work 2021: A Global Workforce View.' ADP Research Institute. https://www.adpri.org/assets/people-at-work-2021-a-global-workforce-view/.

RNZ (2021). 'I'm Gutted, I Didn't Want to Do It.' *Radio New Zealand*, 16 September. https://www.rnz.co.nz/news/national/451610/i-m-gutted-i-didn-t-want-to-do-it-shaw-on-climate-plan-delay.

Roberts, S. (2020). 'COVID-19: The Controversial Role of Big Tech in Digital Surveillance.' London School of Economics. https://blogs.lse.ac.uk/businessreview/2020/04/25/covid-19-the-controversial-role-of-big-tech-in-digital-surveillance/.

Sardar, Z. (2010). 'Welcome to Postnormal Times.' *Futures* 42(5), 435–44.

Sardar, Z. (2013). *Future: All That Matters*. John Murray.

Sibley, C. et al. (2020). 'Effects of the COVID-19 Pandemic and Nationwide Lockdown on Trust, Attitudes Towards Government, and Wellbeing.' Public Policy Institute, NZ. https://www.auckland.ac.nz/content/dam/uoa/auckland/arts/our-research/research-institutes-centres-groups/ppi/policy-briefings/ppi-briefing-covid.pdf.

Spinney, L. (2020). 'Has COVID Changed the Price of a Life?' *The Guardian*, 14 February. https://www.theguardian.com/world/2021/feb/14/coronavirus-covid-19-cost-price-life.

Spoelstra, S. (2020). 'Coronavirus Has Put Scientists in the Frame Alongside Politicians – and Poses Questions About Leadership.' *The Conversation*, 20 November. https://theconversation.com/coronavirus-has-put-scientists-in-the-frame-alongside-politicians-and-poses-questions-about-leadership-148498.

Spoonley, P., Gluckman, P., Bardsley, A., McIntosh, T., Hunia, R., Johal, S. & Poulton, R. (2020). 'He Oranga Hou: Social Cohesion in a Post-COVID World.' *Koi Tū: The Centre for Informed Futures.* https://informedfutures.org/wp-content/uploads /Social-Cohesion-in-a-Post-Covid-World.pdf.

Stanley, E. & Bradley, T. (2020). 'Pandemic Policing: Preparing a New Pathway for Māori?' *Crime, Media, Culture 17*(1), 53–8.

Steyn, N. et al. (2021). 'Māori and Pacific People in New Zealand Have a Higher Risk of Hospitalisation for COVID-19.' *New Zealand Medical Journal 134*(1538), 28–43.

Thaker, J. (2021). 'More Than 1 in 3 New Zealanders Remain Hesitant or Sceptical About COVID-19 Vaccines. Here's How to Reach Them.' *The Conversation*, 8 March. https://theconversation.com/more-than-1-in-3-new-zealanders-remain -hesitant-or-sceptical-about-covid-19-vaccines-heres-how-to-reach-them-156489.

Tollefson, J. (2021). 'Pivotal Climate Summit Dogged by COVID and Equity Concerns.' *Nature*, 10 September. https://www.nature.com/articles/d41586-021-02465-y.

UNDRR (United Nations Office for Disaster Risk Reduction) (2015). *Sendai Framework for Disaster Risk Reduction 2015-30.* https://www.preventionweb.net/files/43291 _sendaiframeworkfordrren.pdf.

Wecke, I. (2021). 'Conspiracy Theories Aside, There Is Something Fishy About the Great Reset.' *Open Democracy*, 16 August. https://www.opendemocracy.net/en /oureconomy/conspiracy-theories-aside-there-something-fishy-about-great-reset/.

WEF. (2020). 'The Great Reset.' *World Economic Forum.* https://www.weforum.org /focus/the-great-reset.

Weisbach, D. & Sunstein, C. R. (2009). 'Climate Change and Discounting the Future: A Guide for the Perplexed.' *Yale Law & Policy Review 27*(2), 433–58.

The White House. (2021). 'President Biden Announces the Build Back Better Framework.' 28 October. https://www.whitehouse.gov/briefing-room/statements -releases/2021/10/28/president-biden-announces-the-build-back-better-framework/.

White, I. (2021). 'New Zealand's Pandemic Housing Policy Has Baked in Māori Inequality for Generations.' *The Guardian*, 17 September. https://www.theguardian .com/world/commentisfree/2021/sep/17/new-zealands-pandemic-housing-policy -has-baked-in-maori-inequality-for-generations.

WHO (2021). 'Mental Health Should Be a Right for All.' *World Health Organization.* https://www.euro.who.int/en/media-centre/sections/press-releases/2021/mental -health-should-be-a-human-right-for-all.

Young, N., Kadykalo, A.N., Beaudoin, C., Hackenburg, D.M. & Cooke, S.J. (2021). 'Is the Anthropause a Useful Symbol and Metaphor for Raising Environmental Awareness and Promoting Reform?' *Environmental Conservation 48*, 274–77.

Index

academic productivity 143–5
African Swine Fever (ASF) pandemic 24, 37
Anthropocene 86, 91
archaeological mode 13
architectural mode 13
Argonauts of the Western Pacific (Malinowski) 182
Assembly of First Nations (AFN) 61
Association of South East Asian Nations (ASEAN) 112
Auckland, lockdowns in 183–7
Azmanova, A. 10

'back to normal' frame 199
bats 25
Bauman, Z. 8
'being there' 181–3
Bhabha, Homi K. 86–7
Bhagat Singh and Others vs. The King Emperor 71
Big Ag 32–6
Bjorklund, K. 44
The Black Death 11–12
Bridle, J. 92
Brown, W. 6
'build back better' 198–9

Canada, COVID-19 pandemic in 61–2
    conditions for 69–71
Canadian Institutes of Health Research (CIHR) 61, 78
CanSino 114
capitalism 13, 107–9
    American *vs.* European 108
    Asian forms of 108–9
    core elements of 107
care crisis 139–40

academic productivity 143–5
domestic labour during lockdown 140–43
cascading disaster 95
case studies 158–69
    creative writing workshops 166–9
    digital photo diary method 158–62
    qualitative social media analysis 163–5
China 109
    Communist Party 113
    Confucian-influenced state 111–13
    economic tensions between United States and 105–6
    and great power cooperation on global health 116–17
    regional superiority 110
    state capitalism 109–13
    tributary system of relations 110–11
    vaccine diplomacy 113–16
civil defense drills 23
Clark, M. 158–62
Coalition for Epidemic Preparedness Innovations (CEPI) 114
coloniality, in Sweden 50–51
colour blindness 54–5
Coming of Age in Samoa (Mead) 182
Commission on Population 52
communication, about COVID-19 pandemic 2
Communist Party of China 113
Confucianism 110, 111–13
consecutive disasters 95
Constitution Act, 1867 68
containment 38
Contribution Agreement 67–8
The Conversation (O'Shea) 44
coordinated market economy 108